Keto Breakfast for Women

2 Books in 1

The Complete Guide To Start The Day With a Delicious Breakfast For All Women With Healthy and Tasty Recipes To Lose Weight, Reverse Aging and Speed Up Metabolism

By

Sofia Wilson

Table of Contents

HEALTHY KETO SMOOTHIES

Keto for Women

Your Essential Guide To Living The Keto Diet With Low-Carb, High-Fat Recipes For Busy Women

By

Sofia Wilson

Introduction

Congratulations on purchasing Keto for women: The ultimate beginners guide to know your food needs, weight loss, diabetes prevention and boundless energy with high-fat ketogenic diet recipes and thank you for doing so.

The following chapters will provide you all the necessary information, facts and scientific explanations that you need to know and master the keto diet. You will find the details explanation on what is the keto diet based on, what are the ketones, what happens in your body when you go keto, how the ketogenic diet will heal and improve many of the processes and organs of your body, how the ketogenic diet is pretty good for people who suffer from diabetes, polycystic ovaries syndrome, seizures, and Alzheimer, the special benefits of the ketogenic diet on women, how it reduces and prevents age-related conditions and many other important and interesting information.

If you came here it is because you are interested in changing your feeding plans, your habits, your body, your lifestyle, and many other things. Let us tell you that you came to the right place. We want to warn you that this might be a difficult process, some of the things written here may not work equally for you than it did for someone else, so we want to ask you to go and see a specialist before making any change to your alimentation

There are plenty of books on this subject on the market, thanks again for choosing this one! Every effort was made to ensure it is full of as much useful information as possible, please enjoy it!

Chapter 1:

What Is The Ketogenic Diet?

The Keto or ketogenic diet consists mainly of the ingestion of 75% fats, 20% high-value biological protein and 5% low glycemic index carbohydrates. That percentage should be applied to every meal. People who want to start with this diet must understand that this is not a diet, but this is a whole new lifestyle and it should be taken as it.

We want to mention that this type of diet has years in the market and has been subject of research on many occasions, demonstrating, in all cases, the wonderful benefits it has on health. This feeding plan is not only for adults; children and teenagers could also use it; so it is highly recommended.

The Keto diet has its beginnings near the 1920s and was made specially as a treatment for the people who suffered from seizures. Over time, and after a lot of researches and studies, the diet surprisingly showed results that were really satisfactory. The first case that possibly has been registered and in which the ketogenic diet for epileptic patients was applied was in 1911. The investigation was led by two French doctors who were Gulep and Marie. They treated approximately 20 persons, between children and adults. The objective of the investigation was to apply this type of diet, added to other protocols known as intermittent fasting.

The ketogenic diet is also very popularly known to lose weight, and lower blood sugar levels considerably, but it is important to know that sugar, gluten and other components that are not within the food permitted in this diet or method of ketogenic nutrition must be eliminated.

As we mentioned above, the major part of the food that we are going to consume is healthy fats, such as avocado, bacon, and peanuts, to mention some of them. In the following chapters of this book, you will be able to see some recipes or plans that you can apply in this diet.

The objective we want to achieve applying the keto diet is to reach a metabolic state in which ketones are the primary energy source of our body. This is achieved by following the diet regularly, with commitment and discipline.

This diet is not based on dietary restrictions, but on significant changes in lifestyle and eating habits, in which we are going to eliminate from our menu processed foods based on refined flours, sugar, and soft drinks. It is a diet that manages to heal marvelously and allow adequate cellular regeneration; Therefore, it improves and even eliminates some diseases, if applied in an evaluated manner with a specialist.

And these changes in the organism are due to the fact that this feeding method gives us the adequate tools for the best functioning of the cellular environment on our organism, and it does so by providing amino acids, essential fats for our body, vitamins, and minerals. This diet is amazing since it doesn't just allow you to lose weight but also makes you feel energy levels that you haven't before.

Any diet can be ketogenic if their bases are respected and if we have the knowledge of cellular processes and metabolism. Diets that can be considered ketogenic are those that force our body to use fats as a source of energy. Fasting can be considered ketogenical since by spending so many hours without eating, the body runs out of glucose and start to use ketones instead. Known this, we can say that a diet in which the lack of carbohydrates is replaced with other foods that has high contents of nutrients can be a ketogenic diet

The main objective of the ketogenic diet is to make our body to get into ketosis, lowering or decreasing to only 5% the intake of carbohydrates. This is a diet low in carbohydrates, and rich in fats that have been compared several times with the Atkins diet and other low-carbohydrate diets, so we share the idea that any diet where these percentages of food are distributed in similar amounts are ketogenic diets, or as it is abbreviated keto diets.

When we start with the ketogenic diet, we decrease the consumption of carbohydrates and replace them with healthy fats. Once this is done, the body will reach or get into a metabolic state called ketosis. In this state, the body is going to become incredibly efficient, transforming the fats in our body into energy. This process will also convert the accumulated fat in our body into ketones, hence supplying the brain with more energy. It should be noted that this eating plan generates higher energy levels than the ones generated by the usual feeding methods.

There are some foods that should be avoided when we are implementing this diet; Some of them are the following:

- Foods with high levels of sugar such as soft drinks, candies, fruit juices, cakes (in this case we would be talking about cakes made with refined flour), and other sweets.
- Foods that are derived from wheat like rice, pasta, cereals or starches.
- Some fruits should be eliminated due to their high amount of sugars. The only fruits that will be allowed are small proportions of forest fruits such as strawberries, blackberries, kiwi.
- The vegetables or legumes. Within this classification are: sweet potatoes, carrots, cassava, among others
- Lentils, chickpeas, beans or legumes.
- Some types of sauces. We would have to evaluate their preparation, as well as the condiments to use. In the keto diet, it is widely recommended to use natural condiments and sea salt mainly.
- Saturated fats are eliminated from this plan. The intake of refined oils, like margarine, mayonnaise, etc. is restricted or limited.
- Alcohol consumption is reduced. As it has high sugar and carbohydrate content. There are some drinks that are allowed in regulated portions and in small quantities.
- The dietetic foods are eliminated preferably; since in their majority and according to several studies, they have a high content of sugar. We recommend that you read very well the labels of the products that you are

consuming, as the majority of these dietetic products are more harmful than the regular ones.

Similarly, there are many foods that can be consumed in the keto diet, most of these foods have a high content of nutrients and vitamins that restore the proper functioning of each of our organs.

As you enter this world, you will know which types of food can help you and bring certain benefits to specific organs. For example, a vegetable that is widely consumed in the keto diet is spinach. This vegetable has a high magnesium content that helps, among other things, to eliminate fatigue and it is a vital food for the brain. Just like the spinach, there are many other superfoods that, if applying this system of conscious feeding, you will get to know gradually.

Among the foods that we can consume are the following:

- The vegetables low in carbohydrates. Preferably it is recommended to consume in higher proportions green vegetables, but you can also eat onion, green onion, tomato, bell peppers, and others
- Fish. Such as salmon, tuna, sea bass, and a wide range of fish.
- Meats are also allowed either red meat, ham, bacon, chops, pork, etc..
- Eggs are widely allowed.
- Butter and creams are allowed, preferably those made with organic materials or milk from grass-fed animals are recommended.
- Cheeses are also allowed. However, the cheeses that are processed are suppressed, by which it is recommended to consume mozzarella cheese, goat cheese, blue cheese, etc...
- Healthy oils such as extra virgin olive oil and coconut oil are very commonly used as well as avocado oil.
- The condiments made naturally. Preferably it is recommended to use sea salt and Himalayan salt, also to season with green natural vegetables like green onion, and coriander, for example.
- It is advisable to consume water. In any feeding plan, the consumption of water is required for the good functioning of the intestine, and the organism in general.

- Last but not least, nuts. They must be consumed in a moderate way. The nuts that you can eat are flax seeds, almonds, walnuts, pumpkin seeds, and chia seeds.

As you have been able to observe, the ketogenic diet is strict and must be followed carefully if you want your metabolism to enter into ketosis. When this food plan is used to eliminate a disease or improve the health of a patient it is necessary to follow it strictly and rigorously so that the body can feed on energy from ketones.

Perhaps, the first few days will be complicated, but once you go through the process called keto-adaptation, you will see the wonderful benefits of practicing this diet, where you will not feel in any way the need to consume processed products, in fact, there are reports and studies that indicate that a person who reaches ketosis can fast intermittently or not with great ease because he has an inexhaustible source of energy due to the ketones produced.

The ketones as you will see in the next chapter, are an inexhaustible source of energy for the whole organism and in greater proportion for the brain. All of our organs consume a certain amount of energy, when we eat, we do not eat to provide calories to our body, but to provide energy to our organs so that each one of them can continue working correctly. And that is exactly what we want to achieve when we feed ourselves ketogenically.

Chapter 2:

What Are Ketones?

This is a concept that comes from the organic chemistry that is seen in high school. It is an organic compound, formed by a group of carbonyls attached to two carbon atoms. The first thing we are going to do is define what a carbonyl functional group is. It consists of a carbon atom that connects, so to speak, with a double bond to an oxygen atom. This type of group is obtained in soda water or blood, as you will expect. The same one is connected with two organic radicals, therefore, we can say that two free bonds are connected to the carbonyl group. These chemical connections are the ones that allow us to differentiate carboxylic acids from aldehydes, alcohols, and ethers. Ketones can be considered less reactive than aldehydes and other organic compounds.

As previously explained, ketones have a similar structure to aldehydes, since both have the carbonyl group. However, the biggest difference between them is that they contain two organic groups instead of hydrogens.

As expected, there are different types of ketones, which are divided according to:

- The structure of their chain: They can be differentiated by the structure of the chain, they can be aliphatic, because the two organic groups that are connected with their carbonyl group, have the structure of the alkyl.

- The symmetry of their radicals: This classification is used when studying the radicals, which are connected to the carbonyl group. When they are the same, as you would expect, can be called symmetrical ketones, but in the case that both are different, they are called asymmetrical, being these the most common in chemistry.

- The saturation of its radicals: Finally, another method of classification. It will depend on the saturation of its carbon chains; if they have the structure of alkenes, the ketone will be unsaturated, on the other hand, if they have the structure of alkanes, it will be called saturated ketone.

There is another type of ketone but is not characterized by any of the three previous classifications. These are called diketones because they have within their chains, two carbonyl groups in their structure. As we mentioned above, these groups are the connection of a carbon atom with an oxygen, connected by two covalent bonds.

Now, to get a little deeper into this subject, let's take a look at some properties of ketones, both chemical and physical:

Physical: Mainly, we can observe that the boiling point of these substances is much lower than alcohol's and have the same molecular weight. As for aldehydes, they do not have a big difference in their boiling point, but both have the same molecular weight.

On the other hand, ketones are soluble in water, but as the chain becomes more complex, solubility decreases.

Regarding the smell, ketones that have a small size, have a pleasant smell, medium size has a strong and unpleasant smell. Finally, the bigger ketones are odorless.

The physical state will depend on the number of carbon they possess since ketones with less than ten carbons are liquid, but those with more are solid.

Chemical: In this case, we have many more properties than in the physical ones. They are:

- Its acidity. Thanks to its carbonyl group, ketones are acid.
- Another noticeable characteristic of the ketones is their reactivity. Ketones are widely used as a product that can synthesize other compounds. For this reason, ketones can be used to make the addition of alcohol, producing hemiacetals, which are not very stable. Another addition that can be made is with ammonia and some of its derivatives, forming a group of substances called imines, which are also chemically unstable.
- They are less reactive than aldehydes.
- Ketones are difficult to oxidize and this can only be achieved with strong elements such as potassium, to say one, thus producing an acid.

Now that we have explained what a ketone is and some of its properties, we can start the book as it should be done.

As you can imagine, ketones are widely used both in industry and in everyday life. We can often find them in perfumes and paints since they are responsible for stabilizing these compounds. Sometimes they serve as preservatives because they do not allow some components of the mixture to degrade quickly. Ketones can also be used as solvents for paints and textiles, in addition to this, they are used in the pharmaceutical industry as well as in those factories that manufacture explosives.

The first thing we must ask ourselves is where to find them in nature. They are found in a lot of places such as human cortisol hormones, testosterone, progesterone, fructose, among others.

It has been proven that some ketones are found in natural sugars in really small amounts, they are found in the fructose, being it a type of sugar. The cells found on the fructose are called ketoses, which can be found on fruits and honey. Although they are ketones, the consumption of them is not recommended for the ketogenic regime, since the concentration of ketones is so small that we will not get benefit of them.

One of the functions that can be done by ketones is the biosynthesis of fatty acids; being this the purpose of the book. What is wanted with this diet is that, through ketosis, a better burning of fats is achieved. In this case, these ketones are generated due to the excessive production of the acetic enzyme. Then, the process of generating the ketone is activated, thus making the cell spread throughout the body thanks to the circulation and goes to the vital organs, such as kidney, muscles or even the brain.

But talking specifically of ketones and what they can do inside our bodies is shocking. The first thing that is done is to release the ketones when the body takes fats instead of carbohydrates as a source of energy. This manages to burn a large amount of fat. That is one of the reasons why in some diets is preferred the consumption of fat than carbohydrates. But, what does this generates?

Levels of glucose in the blood are reduced because carbohydrates become sugar for our body.

In our body, ketones have the function of burning fat to generate energy. For that reason, we recommend diets high in fats and low in carbohydrates; to force our body to generate ketones capable of generating energy. Because in the case that there is a high consumption of carbohydrates, the body will be forced to generate energy through glucose.

Since you know that ketones are cells that you need in your body, you should also guess that there should be a normal or average amount of such cells. By this, we mean that there is a level of ketones in our body which is considered "normal", as is done with other cells, such as white blood cells for example. Therefore, among the levels of ketones in the blood, are the following:

1. Less than 0.5 mmol/L: this means that there are normal levels in the blood. This level corresponds to people who have a diet that fits in normal, regarding the consumption of carbohydrates, fats, lactic, etc.. But what does this mean? Well, that the main source of energy of these people is fructose, or better said, carbohydrates, which implies that fat is not being burned, or not thanks to ketones.

2. The ketone's level in blood between 0.5 and 1.5 mmol/L: this level means small ketosis or mild ketosis. With these levels in blood, it is possible to generate energy through the process of burning fat. Nonetheless, if your goal is to lose weight, it is not yet at the appropriate level. Therefore, this level allows you to control the weight of the person.

3. The level of ketones in blood between 1.5 mmol/L and 3 mmol/L: By having this concentration of ketones in the blood we can consider that we are at the optimal level of ketosis in our body. Being this the level sought by people who make ketogenic diets. At this point, we can take advantage of the ketogenic level. Hence it is recommended to increase both physical and mental activities, in order to get the higher benefits of the keto. When this concentration of ketones is reached, our body will have a better condition to burn fat in an extremely efficient way, thus achieving weight loss.

4. The level of concentration of ketones in blood between 3 mmol/L and 8mmol/L: It is no longer good for the body since the objectives of the ketogenic diet are exceeded. At this

5. point, the results of it are not very positive because it does not have the same efficiency of using fat to generate energy. This level indicates that the body is not functioning properly. For example, the body is not sufficiently hydrated. For people who have a disease, such as type 1 diabetes, the problem may be linked to blood glucose and should be taken into account the level of insulin in their body.

6. The concentration of ketones in blood exceeds 8 mmol/L: This level is alarming since the level of concentration is extremely high for any human being. These values are not due to any ketogenic diet. These cases are found in patients with type 1 diabetes that are not controlled, being its main cause the low levels of insulin. In this case, it can be considered that the patient is in ketoacidosis due to a large amount of ketones in the blood, thus causing vomiting, nausea, and some other symptoms. This situation requires immediate medical treatment.

Already observing all the importance that ketones have in our bodies, we can say that they play a fundamental role in it. The ketones we are interested in are those generated by the liver after the decomposition of fat. But of course, this only happens at the time that the body does not have enough glucose to produce energy from it.

Chapter 3:

What Happens To Your Body When You Go Keto?

By applying the ketogenic diet as a lifestyle, our body goes into a metabolic state that is called ketosis in which our organism feeds entirely on fats.

Ketosis is nothing more than a state in which our body produces large amounts of substances, which function as a source of energy once carbohydrates are eliminated from our diet.

This could be seen as a state in which our organism guarantees its own survival without carbohydrates, learning to use fat as energy in the absence of the glucose substance. In this way our body, mainly our brain not only uses the fat stored in the blood but also feeds on the fats we eat in our food.

Differences Between Ketosis And Ketoacidosis

It is very important not to confuse the state of ketosis with the state of ketoacidosis. The second one occurs when in our organism there are excesses of ketone molecules, and the body is unable to eliminate them through urine, making our organism enter a metabolic acidity that could be considered very severe and even fatal.

Ketoacidosis could be a very frequent risk that all those who suffer from diabetes disease could suffer, being fatal for their organism if it is not treated correctly.

Benefits Of Ketosis

This condition allows our body to access fats found mainly in our bloodstream and the rest of the body. That is why it could be considered an effective way to lose weight.

Ketosis, in addition to allowing us to burn fat faster, gives us a feeling of satiety, reducing our appetite in a considerable way. In this sense, ketosis can help prevent cardiovascular disease.

- The brain: Containing high-fat substances, this provides certain curative properties for diseases such as epilepsy and even neurodegenerative diseases. Besides, has a great impact on the mood.

- In some cases, ketosis can influence diseases such as diabetes.

- Skin improvements related to the acne can be observed, as these ketone substances function as anti-inflammatory for the body.

- It can improve polycystic ovary syndrome and even fertility problems. By avoiding large intakes of insulin, the body increases androgen hormones (especially testosterone) thus increasing fertility.

- The ketogenic diet can improve glucose metabolism by lowering levels of sugar in our bloodstream and may even improve blood pressure and glycaemic profile.

- Ketonic molecules by activating our lipolytic metabolism effectively increases antioxidants in our body.

- Brain injuries: Studies reveal that this type of diet is capable of reducing some brain injuries that have been suffered as a result of an accident causing a more effective recovery in the patient. Many studies conclude that it can benefit Parkinson's and cancer patients, helping to treat some light types of these diseases and reducing the growth of cancerous tumors.

Risks Of Ketosis

Ketosis despite having its great advantages also has some side effects. That is why before starting a ketogenic diet (or any other type of diet) you should go to a specialist to examine your physical conditions and help you to develop a meal plan that can fit your needs. In this way, you will be preventing certain side effects such as:

- Sweating with a strong odor: This happens when ketone cells are eliminated.

- Bad Breath: By having excess of ketone molecules, these will be released through our breath. In the case of suffering this effect, it is recommended to consume a lot of water in order to reduce it.

- Headache: This can happen while our body adapts to our new food routine since our brain will need glycogen for its functioning. We could even feel dizziness.

- Urine with an intense odor: This happens once the ketone bodies are eliminated through the urine, which is why its odor and color can become strong.

- Lack of appetite: By decreasing carbohydrates and increasing protein and fat, our body changes the way it digests food. So we might notice that our appetite is decreasing as our body is getting used to this lifestyle.

- Arrhythmias: When so many changes take place in our organism, it is possible to show some cardiac problems.

Due to the changes that our organism suffers, it is very common that vomiting, decay, nausea, and even respiratory difficulty occur.

By reducing the consumption of fiber such as grains and cereals, we could present constipation.

Usually, this type of diet is not recommended for a period longer than three months because we could feel constantly tired and even lower our performance in everyday activities.

If we want to go back to the nutritional regime we used to have, it is important to follow the same steps we followed to start with the ketogenic diet. We must go back to carbohydrates gradually because a drastic change could cause problems such as sudden weight gain.

Chapter 4:

Heal Your Body

Everybody knows that people who make this diet seeks to lose weight. But it is also used to control some diseases. For those reasons it is important this chapter, that will talk about health.

At first, we want to give a small concept of what health is. According to the world health organization, it is "A state of complete physical, mental and social well-being, and not merely the absence of illness or injury", therefore we can say that health does not mean the absence of any disease. Instead, it means having a certain quality of life that allows us to live in a comfortable way and without so many worries. It is also contemplated to be in a good mental and social state because there are people that you may know who are physically healthy but always feel bad or are depressed. That type of person cannot be considered completely healthy, and in the long run, this has implications on their physical health.

Moreover, a small example of the implications that mental health has with physical wellness is stress because it can affect our health without us realizing. There are occasions in which we get extremely strong headaches caused by anxiety or pain. Sometimes we get muscle tension thanks to restlessness. Chest pain could be for lack of motivation or much pressure; fatigue is due many times thanks to feeling overwhelmed. Changes in sexual desire has implications with anger. Stomach discomfort can be linked to depression. Even sleep problems can be linked to all the previous problems. In addition, it has been proven that diseases such as cancer are often developed by the moods that people have, and also that the happier or mentally healthy the patient is, the better his recovery from disease is. For this reason, it is important to have good mental health, because no matter what we achieve with the ketogenic diet if we are going to have problems with our mental health.

Now that the topic of integral health is over, we can now fully focus on the benefits that keto diet has on our health.

The first thing to do is to reduce the consumption of carbohydrates, sugars and harmful fats, which affects our body for different reasons. The first two foods mentioned, become glucose and if you make a very high consumption of them; they could lead to diabetes. This does not mean that you can not consume carbohydrates, because they are one of the main responsible for energizing our body. The organs, for some of their vital functions, use the glucose into which carbohydrates are converted and thus generate many processes extremely necessary for our body. One of these processes can be when an athlete lifts weights. The muscle will need to use glucose to be able to grow or to synthesize the exercise done; but if the muscles are not able to find glucose in our body, the muscle will decrease in size, in other words, reducing body mass.

Our organs do other processes that need glucose. Nevertheless, that component can be substituted in order to do these vital functions. It is substituted by the ketones produced by the liver. An organ that satisfies these characteristics is the brain since its vital functions can be performed with ketones instead of glucose. A better example could be the previous one; muscles need glucose in order to process the exercise done. This process cannot be done by any other cell other than glucose, but if we are under the keto regime, some organ will have to donate its glucose and feed on ketones. This can be done by the brain as it is able to use ketones to perform its tasks, managing to give energy to muscles to perform their synthesis processes and not to lose muscle mass.

As you can see, glucose consumption is reduced, which means a substantial improvement in the case of people who suffers diabetes since there are some cases in which the patient can stop consuming insulin. There are also cases in which cancer patients were benefited. It is because cancer cells eat mostly glucose cells. Therefore, when eating ketogenically, the production of glucose is reduced, hence the cancer cells are unable to feed themselves. There are also some studies that reveal that the consumption of food recommended by the ketogenic diet helps patients when it comes to receiving chemotherapy or radiotherapy. Although the results are not yet conclusive, it can be said that the results obtained with the ketogenic diet are hopeful.

It is important to mention that it helps reducing overweight. Ketogenic diet's goal is to process fat and use it as energy. Therefore, when burning fat, we can lose weight, then you can lower the rates of overweight, being this one of the most common diseases in the United States and around the world.

When it comes to the brain, the keto diet is also remarkable. Thanks to the keto diet, some of the brain's functions have a better performance. First of all, it protects the brain function. According to studies, it has been discovered that the ketogenic diet could regenerate the in some occasions brain damage. These results were obtained after having done experiments on animals. The first that was done was to feed very old animals with the ketogenic diet. After some time, it could be observed that those animals who fed normally had more difficulty to perform different activities than the ones that were on the keto diet. Then, we can say that the brain works better with the ketones produced by the liver than with the glucose generated by eating carbohydrates or sugars.

At first sight, this diet can be seen as one of the bunch, which has the purpose of considerably reducing people's weight. That idea cannot be further from reality since its health benefits are incalculable. To tell one of the many benefits of keto we will go back to its beginnings. It was used in patients who suffered from epilepsy diseases; epilepsy is an electrical overactivity in some areas of the brain. There were cases in which the children did not respond correctly to the pills that were responsible for controlling the attacks. The solution was the keto diet. Amazing results were obtained as more than 10% of the children to whom this diet was prescribed stopped seizures while more than 100% of the people who suffered from epilepsy and used keto diet could reduce their seizure frequency to about half.

That was not magic, it was because this diet had very important implications related to epilepsy. When the body enters into the state of ketosis, the behavior of some genes of the brain are altered; some of them are responsible for making the energetic metabolism of the brain, thus causing seizures. Another extremely important result is that an abysmal improvement in the energy of the neurons found in the hippocampus could be observed; increasing the density of mitochondria found within the hippocampus.

As if this were not enough, it could also improve the condition of other patients who suffer from Alzheimer's, which is a degenerative disease. This disease will gradually damage the connections that occur in the brain. It affects people in a very tough way since they will lose their memory to the point of not being able to perform their daily or basic activities. But using the ketogenic diet, some of these conditions could be improved.

We cannot say that this stops or reverts the condition, but we can say that there are hopeful results when using this diet in those cases. Experimentations on animals have been made and some kind of healing and improvement were observed on their brains. Even some damage was reverted. This happens because when you enter the ketogenic state, it is possible to reactivate certain neurons and repair part of the brain damage. Additionally, we can see that it also takes care of the brain protecting the dendrites and axons improving a vital process. Dendrites and axons are in charge of brain connections so that the human body can make synapses.

Therefore, we can be sure that the ketogenic diet is not only able to make people lose weight but also allows them to upgrade their living conditions. If the patient suffers any kind of diseases such as cancer or diabetes, we can recommend to try the keto diet, obviously, with the help of an expert.

Chapter 5:

Is Keto For You?

Before trying any diet we suggest to investigate thoroughly in order to understand the consequences that it could have on our body. It is essential to know its fundamentals, advantages, and disadvantages.

It is crucial in order to know if a diet is suitable for our system or not. Because diets works differently for each person.

It is well known that this diet is low in carbohydrates, moderate in protein and high in healthy fat. That distribution is what helps us to reach ketosis; causing the liver to take fatty acids and transform them into ketones to feed itself and use them as energy sources.

This diet is based on a calorie ratio between which 60-75% covers fat intake, 15-30% covers protein intake and 5-10% covers carbohydrate intake.

Among the foods that are allowed in the ketogenic diet, we can mention fats and oils such as almonds, avocado, peanuts, olive oil, fish, pecans, and linseed. It is advisable to eat these proteins that come from an ecological origin such as meats that have been fed on grass, chickens raised in a free environment, fish and seafood, fatty dairy products such as cream, cream cheese, and cured cheeses. Among the recommended carbohydrates are almond butter, mushroom seeds, chocolate (preferably without sugar), consumption of coconut and its derivatives.

The only left step is to take into account the following aspects that could give us a preliminary evaluation to know if the ketogenic diet is convenient for our organism:

1. The keto diet has no restrictions in terms of calorie consumption, so it could be said that we could have freedom with that consumption.

2. The keto diet gives the feeling of being satisfied with meals for longer. This is very good because we do not limit ourselves to reducing our food. Instead, we feed ourselves with what is necessary and we are satisfied with it.

3. The keto diet helps us to have more energy and, although it is known that diets high in carbohydrates generate some kind of energetic decline after eating and that diets low in calories only generate hunger and stress, this diet avoids that by adapting to the fats it eliminates through the reserves and providing us with enough energy to not depend on proteins and carbohydrates. With this, we can have a high energy level during the day and we will not be constantly tired.

In few words, we can say that with the help of the keto diet we contribute to improve our physical quality of life and contribute to our health with long-term effects as long as it is done correctly. All this without worrying about the rebound effect, in which, we lose weight quickly and we gain it back in the same way.

We will achieve this as long as we are willing to radically change our habits. Of course, occasionally we will be able to enjoy a pizza, a hamburger and even cookies at some meal of the day (this must be done very carefully).

The ketogenic diet is not only to feed ourselves in a healthy way, we also must be constant to get a good result. Our body will take its necessary time to process the changes and enter the state of ketosis (may occur within the first 24 hours or up to a week) and be able to begin its process of burning fat and using ketones as energy source.

If you suffer from problems tolerating certain foods high in fat, sugar problems, renal history or any other inconvenience, the ketogenic diet may adapt to your needs, but it is advisable to go to the specialist before making any change in your feeding habits.

It is important to know that ketones do not work the same way as glucose in our body and that is why we need a higher consumption of fatty acids. Doing this, the lack of glucose will be substituted, hence, fulfilling the function of reducing weight, improving our body, eliminating carbohydrates and avoiding the accumulation of useless fat.

It is well known that excess of sugars and carbohydrates are the main cause of obesity, since when fat accumulates it stagnates in our body and can cause serious problems and even have a fatal result in the long term.

All types of diet have their risks and that is why we must be attentive and know if it will fit our body because, otherwise, we can have harmful results.

It is also known that in order to enjoy good health it is important to drink plenty of water and consume varied foods in a balanced way, mostly fruits and vegetables.

Chapter 6:

Benefits Of Ketogenic Diet For Women

In both women and men, the endocrine system is formed by organs and tissues that produce hormones. These hormones are natural chemicals that, after produced, will be secreted into the bloodstream to be used by other organs. It is the general process that our endocrine system performs.

The hormones will then control those organs to which they are destined. However, there are some organic systems that contain their own systems to regulate them without needing hormones.

Now, as women (as this book is aimed for you) get older, there will be particular changes in these hormonal control systems. What is going to happen is that some organs or tissues become sensitive to the hormones that control them, in other cases, the number of hormones that the body can produce decreases with age. Sometimes, it may happen that the hormones decompose or metabolize more slowly.

Knowing roughly what happens with our endocrine system, we can deduce that when endocrine tissue ages, it can produce less amount of hormones than it was likely to, or perhaps it does produce the same amount of hormones but at a slower rate.

Among the hormones that can probably decrease over the years, is the Aldosterone hormone. This hormone is responsible for regulating the balance of liquids and electrolytes in the body. Other hormones are the growth hormone and renin hormone. In women, the levels of estrogen and prolactin generally decrease considerably over the years.

The ketogenic diet induces a metabolic condition that has been called "physiological ketosis" by Hans Krebs and has also been described as an adaptive mechanism preserved within all higher-order organisms to ensure survival during periods of starvation, illness or energy stress.

The ketogenic diet has been used with tremendous success in diseases such as epilepsy. In the case of women, most use it to lose weight and it is due to problems caused mainly by accumulated fat in the body. That accumulated fat has side effects that affect our health, so the main cause of the implementation of this diet nowadays is to lose weight.

When the processes of hyperinsulinism and hormonal alterations are occurring in women, they are not able to ovulate, considering that the entire menstrual cycle is disturbed. This is attributable to a hormonal imbalance between estrogens and progesterone; imbalance that leads to an increase in androgens which destabilizes the entire menstrual cycle and causes women not to ovulate. This increase in androgens starts to affect women's menstruation and other hormonal problems. With the keto diet, these imbalances disappear, actually, there are many gynecologists who recommend it. Surprising results have been seen in women after about ten months of following the keto diet and the evolution and improvement of the "polycystic ovary syndrome".

The entire female hormonal system improves as a result that female hormones are formed from a molecule called "cholesterol". Cholesterol is the basis for the formation of all steroid hormones like glucocorticoids, androgens, estrogens, and progesterone.

This diet is excellent for the liver and the menstrual cycle of women depends directly on hormones meaning that the keto diet helps you significantly for your entire hormonal system. As a consequence that the menstrual cycle is regulated, the ovulation improves, bleeding decreases and in fact, menstrual cramps improve significantly. In the case of women who are in menopause, the diet also helps, now that the production of female hormones is increased. Thus making this stage of the woman's life more bearable.

The keto diet improves brain health, headaches problems, and degenerative diseases. Neurologists are asking women to do the keto diet because, with the reduction of carbohydrates, migraine problems and headaches decrease and, in many cases, it eradicates the disease.

Women also notice changes in their skin such as improvements in acne by cause of reducing processed fats. Improvements have also been observed in skin color, in the decrease of blackheads, and even eye bags. That is why it is currently one of the most implemented diets in the world. All the studies that have been made, based on the diet, show satisfactory results. The life quality of each person who applies it is noticeable and that is why, when you start to apply this nutritional method, you do not want to stop it.

So to finish, we can say that, although it is quite difficult to start this diet and follow each one of the indications as it is really hard to eliminate carbohydrates and sugar from your daily foods, once your body is detoxified from all the anti-nutrients that you have consumed for many years, it will not want to return to consume these foods. When you start with these changes in your habits, your organism will enter into the state known as "keto-adaptation". After that, the changes in your body will start to occur gradually. Do not hesitate on going keto but first talk to a specialist.

Chapter 7:

Using Keto Diet To Control Or Prevent Age-Related Conditions

As the organism ages, it is exposed to different disorders. Those disorders can be both physical and mental depending on each person and their physiology. The changes that occur with age are particularly different according to each person. At the age of 20, it is very likely to have or show diseases or disorders that could be due to congenital or degenerative diseases such as multiple sclerosis, eating disorders that lead, as explained above, to cardiovascular diseases, diabetes, and some others.

From the age of 40 onwards, people tend to suffer from heart diseases and cancer, being those the main cause of deaths. Statistics especially indicate that at these ages the majority of women presents breast and pelvic cancer, and regardless of the genre, skin cancer, cancer of the colon, rectum, and prostate. From the age of 50, it is common to see cases of prostate cancer, as well as obesity, and vision problems. During their 60's, people begin to suffer from bone problems, osteoarthritis, osteoporosis, problems associated with cognitive impairment, Alzheimer's and even Parkinson's disease.

As people get old, if they do not have healthy habits, they are probably going to suffer from one of the diseases or disorders mentioned above. Sugar is an important element in these diseases, as it can alter the cellular environment of our body and thus the destruction or mutation of cells. For that reason, every day there are more and more advertisements that want to encourage citizens to opt for organic food and healthy eating, free of sugars, processed foods, and gluten.

It is difficult to think that after so many years of consuming sugar, now we have to eliminate it from our diet. But if we go back to the past we can remember that our ancestors had longer lives than the actual ones.

Visits and explorations have been made to distant towns in different countries where the entire population has life expectancies of more than a hundred years. When they were questioned about what kind of food they had, the answers were always the same. They fed with the fruits produced by nature, vegetables, tubers, meats, fish, and fruits free of pesticides, gluten, and long-lasting chemicals.

In this context, there are worldwide campaigns to raise awareness of humanity in favor of extending our lives.

The approach of the ketogenic diet goes towards those theories. The fact that we can feed ourselves with food produced by nature sounds incredible. Indeed, physiologically talking, our organism does not need carbohydrates to work, regenerate, nor to survive; neither does need alcohol nor sweets. However, they are the most consumed products these days.

The keto diet eliminates the consumption of processed sugar and this step is important. Positive changes have been observed, such as improvements in disorders coming from age, diabetes, hypertension, polycystic ovaries, Alzheimer's, Parkinson's, and other pathologies.

For this reason, although the most commonly consumed food by humans today are carbohydrates, we must lower their consumption. Their consumption produces glucose in our bloodstream and that energy is not always adequate to feed our body, as it has been observed that when the body feeds on ketones, it is better fed.

In this sense, to have a higher cellular longevity, you should feed ketogenically. This will make your body able to work with the energy produced by ketones. Up to this point, your organism will have burnt accumulated fat from our body

It should be noted that the metabolism changes at around 28 years of age. This is due to hormonal aging and progressive decrease in the production of growth hormone, and the increase in insulin.

Added to this, the food habits that are carried out at present and the lack of exercise accelerates the accumulation of fat and lowers muscle mass. This produces overweight, cellulite, flaccidity, deformities, and so on. As we can see, these hormones are fundamental in the changes produced by age, and the keto diet mainly seeks an increase in the HCG hormone and a decrease and control of insulin.

For example, one of the main problems in older adults is the loss of muscle mass. This happens as a result that the body is no longer able to generate enough glucose; for that reason, the muscles cannot use the same amount of glucose to perform the job of muscle maintenance or the increase in muscle mass when exercising. Then, gradually, due to the lack of glucose generation, the body of older people will lose muscle mass.

That is why making a diet low in carbohydrates and rich in fat, as the keto diet, will modify the way our body works. As there are processes within our body that are done exclusively with the glucose of our blood, others can be done with both ketones and glucose. Muscles use glucose exclusively, but the brain, which is the organ that consumes the most energy can use both. Therefore it consumes the most glucose in a normal food plan, but in the case of a ketogenic food plan, so many ketones are produced that it will feed on them. Because of this, the glucose stored in the bloodstream will be sent to the muscles so that they can maintain body mass.

But we have to be careful with this because we do not want to say that it is impossible to lose muscle mass since there are people who will have very positive results when maintaining muscle mass, but some will not. Saying that all people will react the same to the diet is false.

Something that happens a lot in older adults is the lack of energy. This is because, when reaching a certain age, the body does not work the same way. This can happen either because the body does not secrete the same amount of insulin anymore, so we can't burn all the glucose in our body, generating less energy; or our body does not process the food as it used, generating a lower amount of glucose in the blood that leads to a reduction of energy levels. The solution to those problems could be migrating to another meal plan, in this case, as you might expect, we recommend the ketogenic diet. To lower the consumption of carbohydrates and sugars, and to increase drastically the consumption of fats, will make you able to enter the state of ketosis, thus feeding us through the ketones that could act in a more efficient way in our body. That's why you can hear or see older adults who look very well physically since all this is thanks to food.

Statistically, there have been experiments related to longevity and the keto diet. Hopeful results were obtained, however, experiments have only been made on mice, but it has been shown that their life expectancy increases by thirteen percent due to their high-fat diet compared to those who are fed with carbohydrates. Nonetheless, the most interesting point is not only that they live longer, but they do it better since they do it free of illness and diseases.

Seeing all the benefits that can bring to older adults this type of food we can only recommend you to consume it, of course, always under the supervision of your trusted doctor It can help you to upgrade your energy and thus feel more vitalized. With this, you will have a better functioning of the brain, among other things extremely important for the proper functioning of our body.

Chapter 8:

Supporting Basic Body Systems

When we talk about ketosis, it's just a natural state that occurs when the body feeds mostly on fat when following a low-carbohydrate diet. Ketosis has benefits but also has its possible side effects.

Ketosis is the process where the body produces small energy molecules called ketones, which are known as energy for the body and are used when there is a reduced amount of sugar in blood (glucose). In the human body, specifically in the liver, ketones are produced from fats and then used as energy. The brain does not feed exclusively on glucose, therefore, we can really say that the brain burns carbohydrates when you consume them in the form of glucose, however, if you consume few carbohydrates, the brain will have no problem using ketones instead of carbohydrates. Ketosis is important because the brain consumes a large amount of energy daily, but does not feed directly from fats, it does from ketones.

This function is essential for basic survival, otherwise, as the body stores a supply of glucose product of carbohydrates from one or two days, the brain stops doing its functions after a couple of days without food. After a while, it would have to convert muscle proteins into glucose, but this process is very inefficient to maintain brain function; a situation that would cause the organs to atrophy quickly, due to the absence of food. Luckily, the human body has evolved to be more intelligent, it has fat deposits that can serve to survive several weeks, of course, this being a very extreme case. Anyways, it must be a trained person because not everyone can do it.

When the brain has the opportunity to feed on ketones made from our body fat, many people feel more energy and mental focus, which also accelerates fat burning and in turn, it tries to lose weight.

Ketosis has different benefits that it can provide to the body and the brain; one of the first benefits is to give an unlimited supply of energy, increasing mental and physical performance, and in turn, reducing hunger, facilitating weight loss without so much effort. In addition, in order for the body to enter into ketosis, it is necessary to consume few carbohydrates, effectively correcting type 2 diabetes. Ketosis has been used to control epilepsy and, even without medication, it shows great potential to treat other medical conditions such as acne, and even treat cancer.

For your body to enter into ketosis it is necessary low levels of glucose, since it is our main source of energy. That is going to force our body to look for another food, being it the stored fats in our body. To achieve this, it is essential to follow a strict diet low in carbohydrates as the ketogenic diet. To intensify the ketosis, you can effectively add intermittent fasting.

To recognize if the body is entering into ketosis, it is possible to measure it by a sample of urine, blood or breath. There are also other signs that will be seen without a test; we can say that one of the symptoms is dry mouth and increased thirst and urine.

Keto breath: this means that your body, through the breath, has a smell similar to the nail polish remover; that smell is also felt in the sweat when exercising, most of the time it is temporary. Other indicators but in a positive way, are reduced hunger and increased energy.

As has been said earlier, to achieve a state of ketosis it is necessary to restrict carbohydrates as they become glucose and the body proceeds to use it to energize the brain and other organs. But going fully into the relationship that has ketosis with the body and benefits from it, we can see the following:

- Keto diet and heart: As we all know, the keto diet is capable of making a very considerable loss of weight, resulting in burning fat in industrial quantities. That reduces cardiovascular risks as they often depend on whether the person is obese or also if he has very high blood pressure. As it lowers cholesterol also reduces the chances of having a better protection against heart diseases. Another extremely useful thing about keto diet is that autophagy is increased; it is a way of cellular cleaning, which is great to help our body. Finally, while it is true that it is required to eat few carbohydrates and many fats, it is not recommended to eat bacon every day, but with moderation. The fats that are recommended are the avocado, olive oil, and other sourced of good natural fats that are good for our body.

- Keto and the brain: In addition to the benefits we already know of the ketogenic diet and brain diseases, such as Alzheimer's or epilepsy, we can get other uses of it for the brain such as that it can increase memory capacity. It can be used in older adults or people of any age. It also helps to increase brain capacity because thanks to experiments that were conducted on fat or old animals, with the ketogenic diet they responded better than those who were not fed that way. On the other hand, the ketogenic diet has obtained positive results in people who suffer from congenital hyperinsulinism, which produces hypoglycemia; disease that could cause brain damage. At the time of using this type of feeding, many problems have disappeared in some persons. As if that wasn't enough, it has also been the solution for many patients who suffer from migraines, reducing very often the events of migraine thanks to the low-carbohydrate diet. Patients with Parkinson's have been also benefited from the consumption of the keto diet. These results were seen thanks to some studies that were conducted on this type of patients who were submitted to these diets for at least four weeks. Of those patients, forty-seven percent have reported that they feel better, and the symptoms have decreased. Finally, patients who suffered some brain damage can also visualize an improvement thanks to the ketogenic diet. That improvement attributed to the fact that it is responsible for increasing the connections between the dendrite and axons, which generates better communication between neurons, trying to regenerate the affected area.

Chapter 9:

Diabetes Prevention

Before talking about what might refer to keto in diabetes, it will be necessary to define some concepts.

What Is Diabetes?

It is known that diabetes is a disease in which the level of sugar in blood, also known as glucose, increases disproportionately. This glucose is the main source of energy in our body and comes from the food we eat in our daily meals. Insulin is the hormone produced by the pancreas to help drain that sugar in our blood and thus allow the cells to move in order to function as energy to our body. In the case of diabetic patients, the body is not able to produce insulin and in this way the glucose remains accumulated in the blood, being unable to reach the cells, causing dangerous and even deadly results for the person.

Over time, the excess of glucose in the blood can cause eye damage, damage to the nervous system, and damage to the renal system. It can also cause heart diseases, stroke and patients can even be amputated from a part of their body for damage suffered (due to excess glucose).

Types Of Diabetes

Type 1 Diabetes

This type of diabetes is one in which the body does not produce insulin on its own because of the immune system attacks and destroys the cells that are produced by the pancreas. This disease can appear at any age, but it is mostly diagnosed in children and young adults who must take a certain amount of insulin each day in order to control the sugar levels.

When a person with type 1 diabetes has a low-carbohydrate and high-fat diet, they can stabilize their blood glucose levels. However, this must be monitored constantly as it can cause hypoglycemia.

Type 1 diabetes may be seen as an autoimmune disease (the body destroys itself by mistake). You are at risk for diabetes if you have a family history of type 1 diabetes. This type of diabetes can occur at any age, but it is much more common in childhood.

Type 2 diabetes

This type of diabetes is one in which the body does not produce adequate insulin to control glucose levels. Most type 2 diabetes occurs as a result of a person who has a disordered lifestyle when it comes to food. It can appear at any age, and there are even cases of people who have been diagnosed since childhood.

A person is at risk for type 2 diabetes if he or she has had pre-diabetes or has overweight and does not do any physical activity. This disease is usually diagnosed in people over 40 years of age and in some cases, it is diagnosed in people whose family tree has had this disease.

Gestational diabetes

This type of diabetes occurs in some women during pregnancy and even disappears after childbirth in some cases. However, if a woman has had gestational diabetes, she is much more likely to have type 2 diabetes at some point in her life (either in the short or long term).

A woman is at risk for gestational diabetes if she is overweighted, older than 25, or have a family history of type 2 diabetes. It can also influence if she has the hormonal disorder of polycystic ovary syndrome.

This type of diabetes usually goes away after childbirth, but the baby is more likely to have type 2 diabetes or obesity in his or her lifetime.

As we have been talking about, the ketogenic diet is one that is based on a diet of high fat consumption, moderate protein consumption, and very low carbohydrate consumption. When our body begins to consume glucose that is stored on it, it tries to find a way to get another source of energy, which in this case would be body fat.

This is why it is considered that the ketogenic diet in addition to helping to lose weight, can help regulate glucose levels by taking advantage of excess fat found in the body. Studies have shown that the ketogenic diet can influence up to 60% in the improvement of insulin in the body.

When a person who has diabetes (regardless type 1 or type 2) avoids carbohydrates in his or her dietary routine, which are the main factor in elevating blood sugar levels, he or she may be able to decrease medications to control these levels over time. This is because by not eating food that becomes glucose, the body will be able to respond by its own to insulin.

When starting this diet it is very important to keep track of glucose levels with a specialist, because if the person takes the same dose of insulin (that was medicated before starting the diet) when eating a low-carbohydrate diet, it could cause hypoglycemia which can be very harmful to health.

As we already know, it is not possible for two people suffering from diabetes to have the same dietary approach since they may share disease, but the body's way of reacting of each one is not the same. Ketogenic diets serve the purpose of improving the digestive system by eating healthy as long as it is followed correctly. This will be connected to the patient's physical condition.

There will always be some risks that need to be taken into account if you are under medical treatment. It is very important that under these conditions the patient is fully prepared to assume a diet so demanding that should not have any fault because its consequences can be serious; causing kidney problems, hypoglycemia, ketoacidosis, and kidney diseases. It could be even fatal.

Is The Keto Diet Suitable For People With Diabetes?

Some studies have shown that the keto diet is able to improve the health of some people suffering from this disease and even, in some cases, the minority has been able to improve insulin sensitivity.

Many people see this type of diet as a therapy for the treatment or improvement of the disease; however, this result only applies to some people. Due to the different body types, different patients do not always get the same results.

A person who is not willing to follow such a specialized and strict diet is not going to be able to obtain as goods results as a person who followed this type of diet properly.

What do we mean by that?

Once explained all the factors that influence, you could conclude that the keto diet is highly recommended by experts and people who suffer from diabetes, as they have achieved very positive results in their body and other personal aspects. However, it is very delicate to follow this type of diet, because if you do not have the necessary disposition it could be very dangerous. A slight mistake can damage your health and make a lot of damage.

Can The Keto Diet Prevent Diabetes?

Some studies indicate that the keto diet might, in some way, influence the prevention of this disease (at least as far as type 2 diabetes is concerned) for the person whose purpose is to lead a healthy life. However, many times, this disease is diagnosed from childhood and any type of factor can influence (some failure in the body or possible family inheritance).

Diabetes can be prevented and (if you have it) also controlled up to a point where you will not depend entirely on medications. Of course, this will always depend on the person with the disease and their willingness to change their eating habits.

It is relevant that we are aware that when we make a type of diet in which less than 50 grams of carbohydrates are consumed per day, our body enters the state of ketosis to obtain energy through the burning of fat.

It is crucial for people with type 1 diabetes to be able to differentiate between ketosis and ketoacidosis as the last one can be dangerous because of the lack of insulin. It is also recommended to start with a low-carbohydrate diet in a less strict way (at least 50 grams per day initially) and adapt it to your taste over time.

While people with type 2 diabetes can greatly improve their health condition to such an extent that they can completely overcome the insulin injection, a person with type 1 diabetes will still need to continue injecting their insulin but maybe in a smaller amount.

Chapter 10:
Dietary Exchange Through The Menstrual Cycle

All women possess hormones, which are regulated by three main glands; hypothalamus (located in the center of the brain), pituitary (located in the brain), and adrenal glands (located at the top of the kidneys). These glands are responsible for the rest of the hormones to be in proper balance, thus generating an HPA (hypothalamus pituitary adrenal axis) which is responsible for controlling stress levels, moods, emotions, digestion, the immune system, sexual desire, metabolism, and even our energy levels.

Calorie intake, stress, and physical exercise can cause these hormonal glands to become very sensitive, so it should be considered that a low-carbohydrate diet could affect the body significantly, these changes would be reflected in the attitude.

It is known that long-term stress is capable of generating very serious damage to the body, as the overproduction of cortisol and norepinephrine creates an imbalance in the body that increases the pressure on the hypothalamus and adrenal glands. This pressure causes a dysfunction of the HPA axis.

Referring to adrenal fatigue the most common symptoms that could be seen are fatigue, weakness in the immune system and a very high risk of presenting health problems.

The adrenal fatigue, being a little similar to the suprarenal fatigue has a series of symptoms, between which we can emphasize: fatigue, depressed or weak immune system, possibility of suffering hypothyroidism, inflammation, diabetes, and mood disorders in the long term; being these very serious for the health.

Many times the increase in cortisol levels is thanks to the fact that the person is submitted to a low-carbohydrate diet. As we already know, this is very different in comparison to a moderate-fat diet and for this reason, this type of diet can cause a much greater alteration of stress levels in women than in men.

By consuming few carbohydrates, in addition to generating a noticeable alteration in stress levels, could produce other discomforts such as irregular menstrual cycles or amenorrhea (this means the absence of menstrual cycle for 3 months or more). Amenorrhea is presented by the low levels of many different hormones such as the release of gonadotropin (GNRH) which is responsible for initiating the menstrual cycle and if this failed, would generate a collapse in all (or most) sex hormones, fsh, lh, estrogen, progesterone, and testosterone. Another possible cause of amenorrhea is the low levels of leptin (a hormone produced by fat cells). According to experts, it is mentioned that in women, a certain level of leptin is very necessary to maintain a normal function in the menstrual cycle in order to maintain the regular functioning of reproductive hormones.

Low calorie or carbohydrate intake may cause leptin levels to be completely eliminated, resulting in an irregular menstrual cycle. It is very common for underweight women to be the most vulnerable to low levels of these hormones. Amenorrhea usually appears after a time on a low-carbohydrate diet.

When the keto diet is made, different corporal changes are experienced; but not all of them are always negative. The keto diet could be very useful for those women who suffer from POS (polycystic ovary syndrome), this disorder is the one that suppresses the development of ovaries and the liberation of the ovules. Many of the experimental data indicate that those patients with POS who start the keto diet, manage to recover a regular menstrual cycle and can also contribute to fertility.

When suffering from POS, the excess of insulin in a woman's body is capable of causing a considerable increase in her androgen and testosterone levels, which generates a limitation in the production of estrogens and the body's capacity to ovulate.

When a woman is on the keto diet, she must prepare herself (both physically and psychologically) for the changes she is going to go through.

As mentioned above, it is quite possible that among the changes that may occur is the devastation in the menstrual cycle due to sudden weight loss (caused by alteration of the balance of estrogen and progesterone).

However, an irregular period could not be a worrying change since the menstrual cycle could stop completely; this happens a lot in women who lose a lot of weight and are very thin because their body is more vulnerable to amenorrhea (absence of menstrual cycle) due to anovulation (lack of ovulation).

It is important to note that these problems are very likely to be attributed to sudden weight loss in response to the keto diet. Otherwise, it is very likely due to other factors such as very low body mass index, a low-calorie diet and could even be presented by excess exercise; causing the decrease of some hormones that regulate ovulation, bringing consequences of irregularity.

The lack of carbohydrates could be another key factor in ovulation problems as it directly affects the luteinizing hormone which is released by the brain to help regulate ovulation. When this hormone is directly affected, hypomenorrhea (short, light menstrual cycles) may occur.

Surely you must be wondering... How many carbohydrates must a woman ingest to avoid these types of problems?

It is not really possible to indicate an exact amount since each body assimilates food intake in different ways.

In its majority, the nutritionists indicate to consume between 15 and 30% of carbohydrates, this would be the equivalent to between 75 and 140 grams daily of calories in the form of carbohydrates; nevertheless, there are cases of women in which a diet low in carbohydrates tends to benefit their organism much more (those that suffer from POS).

But, there are cases of women who are recommended to consume between 100 and 150 grams of carbohydrates a day, these can be all those:

- Mothers who are breastfeeding.
- Women who have suffered an interruption of their menstrual cycle.

- Women who wish to gain weight.
- Women who have practiced the Keto diet for a very long time.
- Pregnant women

This type of food intake will be recommended to all those women who suffer from the cases mentioned above; besides, this routine will achieve a harmony in their mood and provide a good amount of energy to perform in their daily activities.

From here, we could conclude that the keto diet can be very useful for those women who suffer from polycystic ovary syndrome which, as mentioned above, is a hormonal disorder that prevents the ovaries from releasing ovules (thus allowing a regular menstruation).

We also know that in some cases women who have made the keto diet, have managed to get a regular period, as well as helping the fertility of women.

Why is this?

This is because, with polycystic ovary syndrome, excess of insulin in the female body increases the levels of androgens and testosterone limiting the production of estrogen and also the ability to ovulate.

In conclusion, the keto diet besides promoting weight loss also helps the symptoms of polycystic ovary syndrome. It is very important to see a specialist before undergoing this diet because, as you could see it can cause a lot of hormonal changes and it is necessary to be prepared for it.

It is also highly recommended not to focus solely on the keto diet but to complement it with another style (as recommended by your specialist). So, in addition to maintaining an ideal weight, it helps you to follow this in the long term and get benefits for your body since the key to a regular menstrual cycle is to follow a diet that adapts to your needs

Chapter 11:

Ketogenic Diet And Fertility

One of the greatest illusions that women have is giving birth to a child. The great majority of women dream about it; they wish to raise him until they are grown up and want to feel proud of them. Unfortunately, not all women are capable of doing that for different reasons, as we will see below, they can be the following:

- Having untreated sexual diseases.

- Having blocked Fallopian tubes. This does not allow sperm to reach the ovule, thus not allowing the stage of gestation.

- Lack of ovulation. If the woman does not generate ovules, then it is not possible to make the union sperm-ovule, which have to unite to generate life.

- Poor quality ovules. This means that they are not able to generate a baby, no matter how many unions are made with the sperm.

- The way in which the uterus is found limits or makes it difficult to have a fertilized ovule.

- Uterine fibroids. Represents having some type of tumors, which are not cancerous, which are like walls or muscle cells, located in the walls of the uterus, they do not allow sperm to reach the ovule.

- Having an endometriosis. Meaning that you get the same tissue that covers the interior of the uterus outside it. We say this, because all the tissue that covers the inside of the uterus, also grows outside it; hence growing in places where it should not; leading to fertility problems.

- Having polycystic ovaries. This indicates that the woman has a disease, which has extremely high levels of hormones specifically androgens. This situation not only affects fertility but also affects the effect of having menstrual irregularities, acne problems and an increase in body hair.

While it is true that the ketogenic diet is not magical and it will not be able to heal all of the conditions it is true that it can help us with one of them; w with the polycystic ovaries. It is important to know perfectly the reason why it helps us and what it is about; since the explanation previously made is very ambiguous or simple. Therefore, it is better to explain it in a better way, so that we are able to talk about it properly.

The first thing is that this is a very common condition in women since it is based on a hormonal disorder in women who are at reproductive age. To start, women who have this condition have extremely irregular menstrual cycles, which can happen rarely or infrequently, or also present a period of menstruation quite long. In addition, generates an excessive level of hormone that is characteristic of men, which is called androgen. Thanks to all these conditions that can be suffered by having polycystic ovaries, small accumulations of liquid start to form. These accumulations can be blood, called follicles in the ovaries that may cause the ovules not to be generated in a normal or regular. Consequently causing fertility problems in women.

The first and very essential thing is to know if you have polycystic ovaries. This is done by observing yourself and verifying if you have a cumulus of symptoms; if you have them, it is recommended to go to a specialist doctor. Fortunately, this condition has treatment which means a great relief for women who have infertility because of the polycystic ovaries.

The first thing we can say is that these symptoms can be seen from the first menstruation happened in the woman. This occurs most of the time, but there is also the possibility that it occurs in an adult stage; nonetheless, the latter may be due to a significant weight gain. But it is important to emphasize that for you to have a real possibility of having polycystic ovarian syndrome, you must show at least two of these symptoms:

- A lot of androgen in your body. This can be seen in different ways, when we talk about the physical form, you can see to have an excess of facial hair or even body hair, but you can also see to have a lack of hair, being it a male pattern.

- Having polycystic ovaries. Which means that your ovaries are dilated, and also could have follicles around your ovules, thus causing a malfunction of the ovaries of women in an age of fertility.
- To have irregular menstrual periods. With this, we mean to present an extra menstruation that is not planned at all with the count of the twenty-eight days in order for the next menstruation to occur. It could also be a very big irregularity in the frequency that each one of your menstruations occurs; being these periods very short or very long. This can be the most common sign for the women who have the syndrome of the polycystic ovaries, this irregularity, could be that a woman has 16 or 7 menstrual periods in a year.

But the syndrome of polycystic ovaries does not appear suddenly, instead, it has some causes, this syndrome has factors which can contribute to deteriorate the situation of the ovaries as follows:

Having excess insulin in the blood: This happens, as you should know because our body is capable of processing the glucose in our body which is the main source of energy if we have a traditional diet high in carbohydrates and the hormone responsible for doing this is insulin; but as long as it is at normal levels in our body. But if this hormone is at a high level, causing the cells to be resistant to insulin, there will be a high level of sugar in the blood, which could cause an increase in androgens in our body thus producing a greater difficulty in ovulation.

Simply excess of androgen, and as we said previously, this causes a very large complication to be able to ovulate, so it becomes almost impossible to have a good fertility.

These causes can also be simply hereditary, therefore, the syndrome of polycystic ovaries can be simply because the woman has inherited this condition from her ancestors.

Little inflammation: this is measured by the production of white blood cells that generates our body, so we can combat an infection. Women who have such a condition have a type of little inflammation that will stimulate the polycystic ovaries which in the long run generate more androgens. Then, in addition to generating hormonal problems, can also generate problems generated with the heart and blood vessels.

When we see the statistics, and we observe the main causes of infertility in women, we can say that eighty percent of them have obesity, but also have insulin resistance and, as we know, having such conditions increases the amounts of androgens in our body. Being insulin resistance the major cause of polycystic ovarian syndrome. In fact, the latest statistics tell us that more than ninety percent of people who have hyperinsulinism, of course in women, have the syndrome of polycystic ovaries, being this a major problem when it comes to the fertilization process.

For this reason, we see that one of the main causes of polycystic ovarian syndrome is having high insulin, the product of having a high level of glucose in the blood and these levels of glucose in our blood are a product of a diet rich in carbohydrates or traditional food. Therefore, by making a considerable decrease in carbohydrates and sugars, we will lose a considerable amount of weight, but it decreases in a more than considerable way the level of glucose in our blood, thus decreasing one of the main causes of the syndrome of polycystic ovaries.

The first thing is that, at the time of losing weight by means of the ketogenic diet, it is possible to reduce in an extremely important way the inflammation. If you were focused enough during this chapter, you could have seen that the inflammation has a direct implication with the process of fertilization because if the woman is inflamed it is possible to get damage in the fallopian tubes, thus causing problems when fertilizing. For this reason, when making the keto diet, we can significantly lower the inflammation within our body, since this type of feeding recommends the consumption of foods that are anti-inflammatory and extremely healthy, thus achieving to lower the inflammation in our organism in such a way that we could unblock, the tube of the fallopian tubes. This will result in achieving an improvement in the possibility of getting pregnant; however, in case of having inflamed fallopian tubes, it is difficult to determine since it does not cause pain, only infertility. Therefore, a way to try to combat this condition is applying this type of diet.

On the other hand, the consumption of a ketogenic diet also allows to have better control of the hormones since the women who possess the syndrome of politic ovaries have a hormonal disorder. This disorder produces a high number of hormones that should be generated by the male gender, causing these problems in the ambit of the ovulation of the woman; for that reason, it is necessary to look for some alternatives to be able to control these hormones.

In this case, the keto diet does not stay behind and allows an exaggerated reduction in the amount of glucose in the blood which makes it possible to control insulin levels. As the person is doing a low consumption of carbohydrates, these glucose cells are not generated, thus achieving the regularization of hormones within the body of females. Moreover, there are specialists in the field that say that a decrease in weight, between five or ten percent, can involve better ovulation. With this, we can say that the ketogenic diet can help regulate hormonal behavior, leading to achieve something so wonderful like healing some women who suffered from infertility problems before doing the ketogenic treatment. There was an experiment that was made with four women, who had the illusion of being able to conceive a child but no matter how hard they tried or how many attempts they made, they had not been able. Surprisingly, after a few months of having started to eat a diet low in carbohydrates, but rich in fat, not only did they lose considerably their weight, but they also managed to rebalance their hormones, helping them to solve some of their infertility problems.

In this case, we can say that these infertility problems can be solved through the ketogenic diet, but by this, we do not mean that it can solve them all, only a few related to the syndrome of polycystic ovaries and overweight. As we have been saying through all the previous chapters, it is never too much to go to the doctor or a specialist to be able to make a treatment in which the woman is able to ovulate or to get to fertilize in order to reach the miracle of life.

Chapter 12:

Basic Recipes

As we know, the keto diet is a low-carbohydrate, high-fat diet plan. Applying this plan will make it possible to reduce weight and improve certain conditions considerably as we discussed before, like blood sugar levels and insulin levels and thus produce a transition in the body's metabolism where carbohydrates will be replaced by fat and ketones.

Now, which are the foods that we must avoid in order to successfully begin this plan?

- Cereals: corn, rice, wheat, barley, oats, grains, sprouts, amaranth, rye, among others.
- Legumes: common bean, chickpea, black bean, green pea lentil, broad bean.
- Starch: potato, carrot, yucca, sweet potato.
- Furtas: banana, papaya, apple, pineapple, orange, grape, mango, tangerine, fruit juices, nuts, fruit syrup, concentrates.
- Alcohol: beer, some wines, cocktails.
- Sugars: honey, agave nectar, maple honey, sugar, corn syrup, fructose, sugar cane.
- The foods that we should consume and that are also recommended in this diet are the following:
- Vegetables: broccoli, cauliflower, spinach, champignons, asparagus, eggplant, zucchini, brussels sprouts, lettuce, paprika, onion, tomato.
- Fats: butter or ghee, lard, homemade mayonnaise, coconut oil, olive oil, cream, dark chocolate, fatty cheeses that melt easily, avocado, nuts and seeds such as flaxseed and chia, almonds, coconut flour, coconut milk, and almond milk.
- Fruits: berries, blackberries, strawberries, blueberries, raspberries.

- Proteins: tuna, ham, chicken, turkey, eggs, sausage, salami, beef, pork, veal, bacon, fish preferably oily fish, duck, and seafood.
- Canned food can be consumed but you will first have to carefully read the ingredients and verify that they do not contain sugars, corn syrup or starch.

Once we have knowledge of the foods we should not eat and those that we should consume we can proceed to know some of the basic keto recipes. In this order of ideas, we are going to proceed to show some short but delicious simple recipes that we can prepare to begin to change our life plan and our diet.

Keto Tortillas With Linseed

Ingredients:

- 300 grams of mozzarella cheese.
- 50 grams of ground linseed, if you have it in seeds you can blend it easily.
- 1 egg.
- Salt to taste.

Steps to follow:

First, we are going to melt the mozzarella cheese (we can do this in the microwave or in a satin). Once the cheese is melted, we are going to add the ground linseed and mix the two ingredients. Finally, we are going to add the egg and the salt. It is necessary to emphasize that everything must be mixed very well so that the tortillas are not left with undesired consistences.

Then, divide the mixture into several portions, depending on the amount that comes out and the number of people, and in a pan over medium heat extend the portions for about five minutes; when cooked, they must be turned with a spatula so that they can cook on the other side.

Keto Tortilla With Almond Flour And Coconut

Ingredients:

- ¾ Cup of almond flour.
- 4 spoonfuls of coconut flour.
- 1 egg.
- Salt to taste.
- 2 spoonfuls of warm water.

Steps to follow:

Place all the ingredients in a bowl, mix and knead until you get a homogeneous dough that is wet to the touch because we do not want it to be liquid to be able to manipulate it.

If we see that the dough is too dry, we can add a little water and knead again and this way you will work with the consistence you want to.

Once you have the dough with the desired consistency, wrap it in a food plastic and let it rest for about 10 minutes.

Once it has rested enough time, we proceed to divide the dough in about eight portions or in the quantity that is wanted, according to the size of the tortillas that are wanted to make.

The tortillas can be given the round shape either with palms with the hands in a natural way or can be made with the tortilla machine or with a bakery roller, if available.

If we make it with the method of the palms, we are going to place the balls of dough in a waxed paper and it will be given the round form with the palms of the hand.

With the machine for tortillas, you will place the ball of dough in the middle with the waxed paper so that it does not stick and crush until you get the tortilla.

Another way is to place the dough balls in the middle of two sheets of wax paper and stretch them with the roller until they acquire the shape, size, and thickness we want.

If we want them to be totally round we can make use of the cutters that are used in pastry.

Later we will proceed to place them in the frying pan (preferably anti-adherent) to medium heat, and let cook for 30 seconds approximately or when we observe that it begins to cook and change color. Then, we turn them to cook on the other side for a few more seconds and so on until you finish the desired amount of tortillas.

EMPANADAS OF KETO MEAT

Ingredients:

For the dough:

- 1 ½ cup almond flour.
- 1 ½ Cup of mozzarella cheese.
- 100 grams of cream cheese.
- 1 egg.

For the Stuffing:

- 1 tablespoon of butter preferably Ghee or clarified.
- ½ Kg of ground beef, you can perfectly mix it with a little pork meat and it will give it a surprising taste.
- 1 tablespoon finely chopped onion.
- ½ chopped tomato.
- Salt to taste.
- Ground pepper to taste.
- Concentrated consommé of beef broth, this is optional to add some more flavor.

Steps to follow:

1. In a frying pan over medium heat add the butter, you can add a little chili if desired, onion, tomato, and let's fry for a few minutes over medium heat until you see that your ingredients are integrating and cooking.

2. Then add the meat, mix, season with salt and pepper to taste, and if we have beef broth, we add it and let all the ingredients cook and mix for about five minutes approximately or until you see that the ingredients are well mixed and cooked.

3. We are going to let the meat cook a little and dry, but not much so that it is a little juicy, then we are going to let it rest to use it to fill the dough and make empanadas.

For the dough:

1. Mix the cream cheese and mozzarella cheese in a bowl, we can melt the cheeses in the microwave or manually in a pot, the important thing is to melt them so they can mix well. After we have mixed the cheeses, we add the egg, mix well to add almond flour gradually, and we are going to mix until a manageable dough is obtained, then let it rest for a few minutes.

2. To make the empanadas we make a few balls, the size will depend on the size we want our empanada. Again, we can make tortillas with the palm of the hands, with the machine to make the tortillas or in its defect with the roller, as explained in the previous recipe.

3. Once the tortilla has been made, add the meat filling that we left to rest earlier. Fold the tortilla in half and seal the dough with the fork so that the filling does not come out.

4. Then place the empanadas in a tray with waxed paper and take it to the oven at 180 Celsius degrees for 15 minutes or until they are golden. And they are ready to taste.

Keto Pizza

Ingredients:

- 200 grams of almond flour.
- 700 grams of grated mozzarella cheese.
- 75 grams of cream cheese.
- 2 eggs.
- 150 grams of salami.
- 150 grams of Pepperoni.
- 150 grams of ground beef.
- 50 grams of Ghee butter.
- 50 ml of unsweetened tomato paste.
- Salt to taste.
- Ground Oregano to taste.
- Garlic powder to taste.

Steps to follow:

1. The first thing we are going to do is preheat the oven to 200 Celsius degrees while we prepare the dough and pizza.
2. For the dough, we are going to melt the cream cheese and half of the mozzarella cheese, we can melt it as it is already known in the microwave or in a pot avoiding of course that the cheese burns. It only has to reach the necessary temperature so that it melts and the two cheeses can be mixed.
3. Once the cheeses are mixed we add the salt to taste, the almond flour, the eggs and we mix everything very well, only in case it is necessary to be able to achieve a better mixture we can place again our container in the microwave to melt the cheeses and to mix well.
4. In a pizza mold, place a waxed paper to prevent our dough to stick; we are going to extend the dough in the pizza mold. A way to extend perfectly the dough is with this technique: we are going to place the dough in the waxed paper and on top, we are going to place another sheet of waxed

paper and stretch. Once reached the desired size remove the waxed paper from above and take the mixture to the oven for about 10 to 15 minutes at a temperature of 200 ºC until we see that it begins to roast a little.

5. For the filling of our pizza, we are going to stir fry the meat with the butter or if we prefer we can do it with olive oil.

6. Once the base of the pizza is golden brown, remove it from the oven and let it rest so that the cheese solidifies, then add the tomato paste mixed with garlic powder and oregano, add the ground beef, pepperoni, sliced salami, and finally the rest of the mozzarella cheese.

7. We put it back into the oven; this time for a few minutes because all we want is to melt the mozzarella cheese, let cool a little and it will be ready to eat. If we want, we can also add olives and mushrooms.

Keto Cream Of Mushrooms With Spinach

Ingredients:

*   1 clove of garlic.
*   ½ Medium onion.
*   250 grams of natural preference sliced mushrooms.
*   1 tablespoon Ghee butter.
*   300 ml of whipping cream.
*   1 cup spinach.
*   1 pinch of salt to taste.

Steps to follow:

1. In a frying pan over medium heat add the butter and cook the finely chopped onion and garlic. When the onion has a transparent color, add the sliced mushrooms and stir constantly so that they do not stick until they are golden and caramelized.

2. Then we will add the whipping cream, the pinch of salt, and move carefully to incorporate until it boils.

3. When the boil breaks, add the spinach, stir and let cook for about two minutes so that the spinach is not overcooked.

4. All we have to do now if we want to; is to blend all the ingredients to obtain the cream. There are people who do not blend it and the flavor is just as wonderful, once the cream is obtained we serve it hot and enjoy.

5. If we get leftover cream, we can refrigerate it in a container with lid and save until the next time we want to consume, at that time, it can be heated in a frying pan over low heat. This recipe can also be used as a sauce to complement a chicken or pork and is equally delicious.

As we can see, it is easy to take this food plan and once we try the recipes we will realize that they are as tasty as the usual diets. It is crucial to try that the food is accompanied by nutrients that our body can absorb, such as spinach and vegetables, coconut oil and other foods that provide a good amount of vitamins and nutrients necessary for our body.

Chapter 13:
Food Choice

It is already known to us that if we eat the right diet we can reach the desired levels of ketosis and enjoy the many benefits that this provides.

That is why it is important to evaluate very well which foods we are going to buy when starting the ketogenic diet. The important thing is to choose products that, in addition to being allowed in the keto diet, provide us with the vitamins and minerals that our body needs because, as the cellular environment is regenerated and cleaned, we will have the ability to absorb all the nutrients from the food ingested.

Based on this, we are going to talk about some foods that are supposed to be consumed in this diet for the nutritional contribution they have for our body. Whitefish, such as hake or similar fish are a good choice as they are lean options and very reduced in calories but with a high-quality protein for our body, especially for its high proportion of omega 3, essential for health.

The avocado is one of the few oily fruits sources of vegetable protein admitted by the keto diet and also widely used in this food plan for its big versatility when preparing a dish as it is used for salads, sauces, and even desserts. The avocado is a fruit considered an excellent antioxidant and rich in vitamins and minerals, with a natural fat that is widely used in these keto diets.

Vegetables are also allowed and widely recommended in the ketogenic diet; especially green vegetables. These green vegetables are source of vitamins and recommended fibers; in the specific case of spinach we have that it is a vegetable used in most keto dishes and it is because spinach, apart from containing fiber, has vitamin A, B1, B2, C, K, calcium, phosphorus, iron, folic acid, is rich in magnesium, zinc, and beta-carotene, the latter slowing the action of free radicals, making spinach to be considered as a natural anticarcinogen. Spinach can improve the functioning of the immune system and vision. As we already know, vegetables form most of the distribution of food that must be present in the daily dishes so it is necessary to ingest products of good quality and with a great contribution such as spinach.

In the case of vegetables, not all vegetables are allowed in the keto diet, this is because some of them have a high content of starch and carbohydrates that are processed by the body as sugar and, as far as we know, we must avoid it in this diet plan. That is the case of the potatoes, sweet potatoes and cassava, for example. However, there are other vegetables that are allowed since they are low in carbohydrates, such as cauliflower, broccoli, bell pepper, celery, cucumber, eggplant, and asparagus. Cauliflower is a highly recommended and used vegetable, low in carbohydrate and high in fiber and vitamin C.

When talking about cheeses, the first thing we are going to recommend is to consume organic and defatted cheeses coming from animals preferably fed with grass. It is important to be able to evaluate the nutritional information of the cheeses that are ingested, the lesser ingredients they have the better they are since there are many products that can have stabilizers that add carbohydrates and sugars to the cheeses.

A topic of discussion is the consumption of milk as it contains large amounts of carbohydrate so the milk allowed is from nuts; such as almond milk, and coconut milk without sugar. The detail is that many specialists do not recommend consuming those milks because to generate a glass of almond milk, it requires large amounts of almonds, thus exceeding the amount of fat you can ingest daily. You consume large amounts, of course, that is what it is recommended in the keto diet, but moderately. The same applies to almond and coconut flours. In the case of clarified butter or Ghee, just like the oils allowed, its content is clearly fat without carbohydrates or proteins. In fact, more than 60% of the ketogenic diet is fat, so they are one of those that can be used with more confidence for the preparation of most dishes. It is recommended, as we have been saying previously, to choose good quality products and, currently, on the market there is a wide variety of them.

Nutritional yeast is a good ally of people who apply the ketogenic diet because when it is sprinkled on meals you get a delicious cheese flavor, it is also rich in vitamin B12 and is often used to make cakes and breads.

Another component of food that we can not leave behind and that we want to recommend is collagen. This can be found in the gelatine extracted from the broth of beef legs, for example. Collagen is the most abundant protein in mammals including humans. It is one of the most important components, especially in these processes in which people are losing weight and reducing sizes and is required to improve the elasticity of the skin. Collagen helps the skin, bones and connective tissues and represents almost a third of our total mass of protein.

That is why we strongly recommend consuming gelatine that is collagen in a natural way. The most commonly used is the gelatine made with beef legs broth, which contains a large amount of collagen protein.

There is an oil used in the ketogenic diet that has many properties and it is the MCT oil, it consists of concentrated caprylic acid and which is 8 times more concentrated than coconut oil.

MCTs are easy to absorb fatty acids that metabolize very quickly and are effectively converted into long-lasting energy for the brain and body, and help to increase energy, endurance, and mental concentration while in a low-carbohydrate or ketogenic state.

MCT oil increases metabolism and improves your body's ability to burn body fat as a fuel source. As MCT oil is naturally tasteless and odorless it can be easily mixed with food without altering its flavors. For those who are starting to consume this type of oil, it is advisable to start with half a teaspoon that can be added to the morning coffee or in the coffee with which you are going to break the fast for example.

The Himalayan Pink Salt is another good recommendation that you can add to the amount of products that you must acquire if you are going to start this diet since it is a salt that preserves all the essential minerals and electrolytes, promotes healthy pH levels in the body, contains natural iodine, improves circulation, and does not increase blood pressure. Otherwise, common salt is not recommended because its minerals are lost in the process of industrialization and it can cause high pressure in the body when consumed in excess; iodine in this type of salt is artificially added in and it also includes anti-glomerate compounds. So when consuming salt in our meals choose pink salt or Himalayan salt.

With all that we have been able to appreciate so far, we have that within the great variety of foods allowed, if we evaluate and investigate their enormous properties and, in addition, we look for different combinations of dishes or menus that we can do with them, we will not find ourselves in the need to get bored of this lifestyle. We have to learn why some vegetables, for example, are not allowed in the food plan, only in this way and acquiring the knowledge about nutritional content of each of the foods we consume, we acquire awareness and responsibility of not consuming it.

Let's talk about cereals. They have a certain quantity of starch, some have more than others, that are metabolized in our body in the form of sugar; something that we should not consume in the keto diet. So, this type of food should be avoided, such as the case of rice, and we can replace it with keto rice using cauliflower. There is a wide variety of options that we can do and try to adjust the plan, not only to our economic needs but also to the needs and requirements of our body.

In the case of alcohol, it is not recommended to consume beer, cocktails and some wines. In the ketogenic diet, some types of wines may be allowed, such as dry wine containing less than 0.5 grams of sugar per glass. Most wines are presentations of beverages with carbohydrate concentrations due to various fermentation processes such as glycerol, which has a minimal effect on blood sugar concentration or insulin levels. With this information, we can use the analogy that every time we consume a glass of wine we are drinking 2 grams of carbohydrates.

When applying the keto diet, if we want to achieve the benefits and be able to obtain the levels of ketosis; we must not only be aware that we must follow the indications of the ketogenic diet, but also have some examples and some knowledge that we must take into account when choosing foods. Knowledge like: which vegetables are not allowed and which are the consequences of their consumption. We must also evaluate which foods we will consume and why, what benefits it would be contributing to my diet. If we do this process in a planned way organizing a weekly menu, for example, we can achieve our goals easily.

As it has been reiterated on several occasions, this type of food should be monitored by a nutritionist or expert in the area because each body reacts differently and the requirements of one person are not the ones of another person. In addition, each person may have different inflammatory problems or food allergy that should be considered before starting any diet. Although the keto diet is wonderful and has a wide variety of proven benefits, it is also true that each person should be evaluated by an expert.

Chapter 14:

Breakfast

When practicing a traditional eating plan (with this we mean one that has a normal intake of carbohydrates) it is said that breakfast is one of the most important meals of the day as people go a long period without eating food from the night of the last day. This implies that this is the first meal of the day; the one that allows people to get enough energy to face their day with all the challenges it can have. If you do not eat breakfast, and then eat lunch, for example, it is very likely that people will feel hungry throughout the day.

For the reasons stated above, it is important to show you some recipes in order to have a good ketogenic breakfast.

Cups Of Egg, Ham, And Cheese

This is a very simple recipe, as you do not need many ingredients. They are cheese, ham, and eggs; these are ingredients that can be found in every fridge. Besides, this is not very complicated to prepare since you do not have to be a chef to make it. In addition, it can also be done very quickly, in an approximate time of twenty-five minutes. So, if you are in a hurry for the daily struggle, this recipe is very good for you. The ingredients are as follows:

- A spoonful of butter.
- Twelve slices of ham.
- A cup of shredded cheddar cheese, or a cheese that is fatty.
- Twelve large eggs.
- Salt to taste.
- Pepper to taste.
- Freshly chopped parsley.

When we see these ingredients, we can see that the recipe does not require anything out of the ordinary. Hence, anyone can make this recipe and as you will see below, it is not a very difficult process.

1. Preheat the oven at 400°.
2. Grease a tray of muffins with butter; you are going to grease the cavities of the muffins.
3. Place the slices of ham inside the muffin cavities covering them with the ham.
4. Place the cheese inside each cavity, above the ham that has already been placed.
5. Break one egg per muffin cavity on top of the cheese.
6. Season with pepper and salt to taste.
7. Decorate with parsley.

By observing how it is prepared, you can see that its preparation is extremely simple, for that reason, you can cook it without the need for having advanced knowledge in the kitchen. All you have to do is to preheat an oven, and then put ham, cheese, and egg; then wait until everything is ready. This recipe is very simple, but at the same time, it is very tasty.

Stuffed Peppers

For this recipe, not much is needed, only bell peppers and eggs. Obviously, you can add the ingredients you want, as long as what you want to add is allowed in the ketogenic diet. This recipe is as simple as the last one, but in this case, instead of using molds for muffins, we will be using the bell peppers.

The ingredients are as follows:
- Two large bell peppers, halved and seeded.
- Eight beaten eggs.
- A quarter of a cup of milk.
- Four strips of bacon, cooked and toasted, cut into small squares.
- One cup shredded cheddar cheese.
- Two tablespoons of scallions, finely chopped.
- Salt to taste.
- Pepper to taste.

As you could see, the recipe doesn't need many ingredients, and the ones you need are very common, therefore, for you to make this breakfast, you don't need many things. If that wasn't enough, the process to cook this breakfast is extremely simple.

1. Preheat the oven at 400°.
2. Place the peppers on a baking tray facing up and add a little water.
3. Put the peppers in the oven for about five minutes.
4. Beat the eggs and milk until smooth.
5. Add bacon pieces, cheese, spring onion, salt and pepper to taste.

6. Pour the mixture into the peppers, and leave them in the oven. Leave about thirty to forty minutes in the oven.

As you can see, this recipe is extremely simple and does not need much more than simple ingredients. This recipe consumes a little more time than the other one, but it is worth it, so we can only recommend you to cook it and try it.

Chapter 15:

Lunch

Lunch is a vital meal for the human being, even despite being in a ketogenic diet, it is always important to eat three meals a day. Skipping one of the three main meals affects the metabolism of each person.

To be able to make such a diet, and not suffering in the attempt, we will recommend you to make the following recipes:

Cobb Egg Salad

Eating salad is always good, for that reason, we recommend you to eat it. It has different foods rich in fats; they are foods such as bacon or avocado that has natural fats which help our body to enter ketosis. The ingredients are as follows.

Ingredients:
- Three tablespoons of mayonnaise, preferably natural.
- Three spoonfuls of Greek yogurt, since it is the healthiest of all.
- Two spoonfuls of red wine.
- Kosher salt.
- Black pepper to taste, as this doesn't affect the ketosis process.

- Eight boiled eggs, you can chop as you wish, it is recommended to chop them into several round pieces for decoration, but if you are a person who does not care about the appearance, chop them as you like. That amount is the minimum, but you can use the amount of boiled eggs you want.
- Eight strips of bacon, which you can cut into strips or squares. At the time of cooking, this amount is recommended as a minimum, but you could consume more bacon, so you can decorate the Cobb egg salad.
- An avocado that should be cut into thin strips. You can cut it as you like either as squares or strips and you can consume the amount of avocado you wish.
- Half a cup of blue cheese shredded or crumbled, this the cheese is not exclusive, you can consume the cheese you want, such as smoked or yellow cheese as long as it is high in fat.
- Half a cup of cherry tomatoes, the same chopped in half. If you do not have this type of tomatoes, you can also eat regular tomatoes, chopped in small squares.
- A quantity of two tablespoons of chives chopped very small.

Now, the preparation process is very simple, only two simple steps are needed.

1. In a small bowl add the mayonnaise, the Greek yogurt, and the red wine, stir well until you have a homogeneous mixture, after having done that, proceed to add salt and pepper. This step is responsible for making the sauce, or rather the salad dressing.
2. Then, in a larger bowl, we proceed to add the eggs, bacon, cheese of your choice and cherry tomatoes; after they are all there we proceed to gradually add the dressing previously made, it is going to be added until all the ingredients are well covered with it, after that, try the salad and proceed to add salt and pepper to taste. Finally, add the chives to decorate the salad to taste.

As you could see, the process and the ingredients to make this salad were really very simple. The preparation should not take more than ten minutes since you only need to chop the vegetables, cook the bacon, make the eggs, and mix well, which should not take much time nor knowledge in the culinary field.

Stuffed Avocados

This is a very simple and fast recipe, for which you do not need many ingredients. All you need are avocados, onions, fatty cheeses, nothing too exotic or very difficult to get because you only need things that you can get in your home market. Besides, you do not need to be a chef since this recipe is extremely simple; on the other hand, if you are in a hurry you won't waste a lot of time either since the time it will take you to prepare this recipe is between ten minutes or a little more. The recipe quantities are equivalent to about four portions for people who do not eat a lot, but for people who are used to eat a lot, could serve as two portions.

The ingredients are the following:
- Four avocados that are well ripe.
- The juice you can get from a lemon.
- A spoonful of olive oil, preferably extra virgin.
- An onion of medium size, which is chopped as you prefer.
- One pound of ground beef.
- Condiments of your preference to prepare the tacos. Moreover, there are packages made for you to prepare the tacos.
- Kosher salt to your liking.
- Black pepper, fresh and freshly ground.
- A cup of yellow cheese, or also Mexican shredded cheese.
- Half a cup of chopped lettuce.
- Small chopped cherry tomatoes, or regular tomatoes chopped in small squares.

- Sour cream, for consistency and decoration.

After having all these ingredients, we can proceed to the preparation but it should be noted that to make this recipe; the ingredients we just mentioned are the basic ones so if you want to add more ingredients you can do so. As long as you do not go out of what stipulates the ketogenic diet, which is not to consume carbohydrates or sugars. Well, explained that point, we will proceed to explain how to make its preparation.

1. We take our avocados and chop them in half, we take out the seed, boning the avocado, thus leaving as a hole in the avocado, which is the space occupied by the seed. Finally, we put lemon juice to our avocados, to prevent them from oxidizing.

2. Then, place in a frying pan over medium heat the oil until it is bubbly, at that time, that the oil is very hot, add the onions that had already been chopped. Let them cook until they are golden, this may take a little bit, about three or five minutes.

3. Add the ground beef and the seasoning of your preference; then, with the help of a wooden spoon, move the meat, also keep seasoning with salt and pepper. Afterward, the beef is going to be put together in the pan with the onions. Cook until the meat is not pink, this meat cooking lasts about five or six minutes.

4. After the meat is cooked, drain the fat from it.

5. After draining the meat, proceed to grab the avocado and fill in the avocado holes with all seasoned ground beef. Finally, at the top of the stuffed avocado, add the cheese, tomato, lettuce, sour cream and enjoy your meal.

As you could see, in order to make the avocado tacos recipe you don't need to be a chef. It only takes a little time, and it's not much since it should take about ten minutes, therefore, this recipe is extremely effective when you are busy or in a hurry. Besides, it will allow you to continue with a keto lifestyle without losing or skipping good meals because practicing this style of food, does not mean eating badly or insipid, it is quite the opposite.

Keto Bacon Sushi

For lovers of Asian food, especially those of sushi, we have this dish, which is not really sushi but it has its form because when preparing it, we will give it the shape of them. It is very similar to the traditional sushi, but a ketogenic one. No special ingredients are needed either, because you can use carrots, bell peppers, among others. It is also important to say that this recipe will also provide a perfect balance, as you will eat vegetables and some fats. The estimated time to make this recipe, adding the time to chop all the ingredients, and then cook them, is half an hour, therefore, although we could see an increase in time when cooking the recipe, we can also see that we are expanding our menu with simple recipes.

The ingredients are as follows:
- Six slices of bacon, the same chopped in half, to then be able to use them to make the covering of the pieces of sushi. The bacon in this recipe will act as the seaweed, which will cover the sushi.
- Two cucumbers, it is recommended that the same are chopped into thin slices.
- Two medium carrots, it is also recommended that the carrots are chopped into very thin slices.
- Four ounces of cream cheese, quite soft, so that after it can be mixed with other things.
- Sesame seeds to decorate.

After having the ingredients chopped and everything ready, we proceed to begin the cooking process, but not before specifying that we can make keto sushi with any vegetable, in this case, we are using carrots, but they can be replaced by bell peppers to say something different than carrots. Now, let's get to work.

1. The first step is to preheat the oven to four hundred Celsius degrees.
2. We take some of our trays, which we use for baking and we will wrap it in aluminum foil.
3. Place the bacon on top of the aluminum that has covered your tray, so that it can be cooked. It must be placed in such a way that the halves of the bacon are in a symmetrical way or better said, place the bacon so as to create a uniform layer. They should be baked until the bacon is crispy but also that a little easy to fold, possessing a certain grade of flexibility.
4. Then cut the carrots, avocados, and cucumbers to the same width as the bacon.
5. After the bacon has rested so that you can touch them with your hands, you will proceed to put a little cream cheese on top of the ends of the bacon and proceed to take the vegetables that you had already chopped and place them evenly on it. Preferably, place those vegetables at the ends of the bacon.
6. Roll up the vegetables quickly and tightly with the bacon.
7. Finally, we proceeded to decorate the recipe with seeds of alamo to the taste of each guest.

As we could see with this recipe, which sounds delicious, you don't need a lot to eat delicious, you just need imagination and a little time. As we said previously, vegetables can be replaced, not only we can make keto sushi with carrots, we can also use tomatoes, bell peppers, cucumbers, among other foods. You just need imagination to make this recipe more diverse and more delicious.

As you could see in this chapter, with these three recipes of ketogenic lunches, you will not lose the quality of your food, only that you will not consume carbohydrates. With this, we mean that your food will not lose flavor. Instead, it will maintain it, therefore, you will not find it difficult to migrate to this type of ketogenic food since as you can imagine, the flavor is delicious and you will be feeding better, cellularly speaking. What we can tell you is to try these recipes, investigate new and different recipes to make variated lunches, and create your own ones.

Chapter 16:

Dinners

Generally, dinner is a dish that is difficult to plan. Perhaps we spend all day in most cases in the street and when we get home we do not want very elaborated or difficult menus. Nevertheless, there will be special occasions in which we will have time to prepare a delicious dinner. For those who practice fasting, probably this is their second meal of the day, for those who don't, we talk about the third meal of the day. Regardless of the case, we must take into account that at the evening meal it is recommended not to consume or reduce to the maximum the consumption of carbohydrates. In this order of ideas, we will give some recipes for dinner following the ketogenic style.

Breasts Stuffed With Pesto Sauce And Mozzarella Cheese

Ingredients:

- 3 breasts
- 250 grams of Mozzarella cheese approximately, if you like a lot of cheese add more.
- A large fresh bunch of basil.
- 1 clove of garlic
- Olive oil to taste
- A handful of almonds
- Shredded Parmesan cheese to taste.
- Salt and pepper to taste

Steps to Follow:

1. Wash the basil leaves well and add them to the glass of the blender. Now add the almonds and the whole peeled clove of garlic. Then add 3 to 4 tablespoons of olive oil, a little salt, and pepper to taste and proceed to blend. We must obtain a creamy emulsion; if we see that it lacks more liquid, we can add more oil until it reaches the point that more pleases us to the palate.
2. We must ensure that everything (especially the garlic) is well crushed.
3. When the sauce is ready, blended, and with the desired consistency, add the Parmesan cheese and, if you want, blend again at medium speed, there are people who do not blend the cheese and can do so as well.
4. Now with this delicious pesto, we are going to fill the breasts.
5. We are going to open the breasts like books, and we are going to add salt and pepper to taste.
6. We add a good and appetizing layer of the pesto we already prepared and later we place several slices of Mozzarella cheese on top.
7. Roll up the breasts and hold them with sticks of wood or bamboo.
8. We can cook them in the oven or in a non-stick frying pan. And the tasty dinner of breasts stuffed with pesto and Parmesan cheese is ready.

Hake With Romesco Sauce And Vegetables

This dish is ideal for the night when you want to make a more elaborate meal. The sauce is ideal to accompany both fish and chicken as the case may be. This recipe is designed to get a thick sauce, you can make it more liquid if you like. Here I use the hake but you can choose the fish you want.

Ingredients:

- 1 ¼ Cup of Almonds
- 2 cloves garlic
- 500 grams of bell peppers
- 3 Tomatoes
- 1 Gren onion
- Half Onion or a medium Onion.
- Olive Oil
- Salt to taste
- Pepper to taste
- 3 Hake

Steps to follow:

1. First, let's make the sauce. Cut the bell peppers into pieces and process them together with the tomato, onion, garlic, and almonds; you have to process them very. We are going to process for about 30 seconds; when we are processing everything we add about three or four tablespoons of olive oil. We see the consistency as we process the mixture. When we say process we mean to cook.

2. When the sauce is ready we proceed to make the hake, once cleaned and filleted we add a little lemon, this step is optional according to the taste of each one, but the seasoning with lemon gives a wonderful aroma and flavor to the fish. Then we are going to season with salt and pepper. And we are going to place them in a frying pan, preferably non-stick, and cook

carefully over medium heat until they are ready. Obviously, we will have to turn them so that they cook on both sides.

3.   Once ready and served, add the romesco sauce on top of the hake.

If you wish, you can accompany it with avocado and stir-fried bacon, it is a wonderful combination for this dish.

Broccoli And Sausage Tortilla

It is a simple dish to make for dinner and within the standards of the ketogenic diet. If you like it you can add more vegetables to it.

Ingredients:

- 1 large whole broccoli.
- 2 or 3 sausages; should be organic chicken, preferably pre-cooked.
- Clarified Butter or Ghee.
- 6 large eggs preferably.
- Fresh oregano, chopped parsley.
- Salt to taste.
- Pepper to taste.
- 1 avocado.

Steps to follow.

1.   The first thing we are going to do is to cook the broccoli. It is recommended to boil the water first in a pot and once the water is boiling we are going to place the broccoli in a period of about 3 to 5 minutes since we do not want it to be overcooked. Actually, it will be better al dente. Once cooked the broccoli, we submerge it in ice water to stop the cooking, and later we chop it in small pieces and add salt to taste.

2.   In a frying pan add ghee butter and the sausages that were previously thinly sliced and cook them. When they are ready, add the broccoli, fry it together with the sausages and add salt, oregano, finely chopped parsley

to taste, and fry it a few more minutes. In a bowl, we are going to pour the eggs and beat them until obtaining a homogeneous mixture.

3. Then in the pan where we have the sausage and broccoli fried, we are going to pour the eggs and let them cook for a few minutes. When we observe that the tortilla is almost done, we remove it carefully from the pan, we take it off and turn it so that it is cooked on the other side for a few more minutes.

4. Once the tortilla is ready we serve it and on top of it, we are going to put the sliced avocado, in addition, if it is of our taste we can sprinkle over it a little salt and pepper to give the final touch.

Chapter 17:

Sweet tooths, snacks and desserts

When starting any diet and mainly the Keto diet, we could feel hungry or anxious at some moments. To avoid that feeling it is advisable to eat some snacks as long as they are carbohydrates-free. This way we can stay in the Keto line.

Let's remember that snacks are mostly a type of light food that we eat when we have anxiety, these in a certain way give us energy. The problem occurs when these snacks are eaten in large quantities and very often, as they are made from heavy ingredients that provide more fat to our body.

There are many ways to calm the anxiety or feeling of hunger with pleasant and healthy options so that we have are not guilty of giving us a taste. Next, we are going to show you a variety of options of snacks approved by experts in keto that will keep us satisfied without leaving the diet.

These recipes could be ideal as a snack or even as a dinner since they do not require much preparation:

- Slice of cheese spread with butter
- Celery stuffed with cream cheese
- Slice of cold butter spread with peanut butter
- Lettuce or cucumber spread with mayonnaise
- Small radishes with butter
- Parmesan cheese fries with butter
- Cheese and salami slices rolled up
- Sliced bacon with peanut butter or butter
- A square of dark chocolate with butter
- One tablespoon of butter or coconut oil melted in tea or coffee

On the other hand, we have a list of snacks a little more elaborated and tasty for those moments of anxiety. Ketogenic snacks are a good option to keep us on the diet in case we feel hungry.

Eggplant French Fries

Ingredients:

- 2 eggplants
- 475 ml (250 g) ground almonds
- 1 tsp cayenne pepper
- Salt and black pepper to taste
- 2 eggs
- 2 tbsp. coconut oil spray

Preparation:

1. Preheat oven to 400°F (200°C).
2. Peel the eggplants and cut into chips. Add salt (a little) on all sides to prevent the eggplant from becoming bitter.
3. In a not very deep bowl, mix the ground almond, cayenne, and pepper, in another bowl add the eggs beating until frothy.
4. Pass the chopped eggplants through the almonds, through the eggs and again through the almonds.
5. Place the eggplants "potatoes" in a baking tray previously greased, sprinkle coconut oil on top.
6. Bake for 15 minutes or until golden brown and crispy.

Bacon And Cheddar Cheese Balls

These balls are not only delicious but also ketogenic, bacon and cheddar cheese are a perfect and delicious combination, here we leave the preparation:

Ingredients:

- 150 g bacon
- 1 tablespoon of butter
- 150 g (150 ml) cream cheese
- 150 g cheddar cheese
- 50 g butter (at room temperature)
- ½ tsp ground black pepper

Preparation:

1. Melt the butter and fry the bacon until golden brown.
2. Remove from the frying pan and let cool on absorbent paper.
3. Cut the bacon into small pieces and place them in a bowl.
4. In another bowl, mix the excess fat from the bacon with the rest of the ingredients.
5. Leave the mixture in the refrigerator for 15 minutes to harden the mixture.
6. Assemble the balls, pass them over the bacon and serve.

Spinach, Artichoke And Cream Cheese Dip

Ingredients:

- 1 cucumber, chopped into sticks
- 2 cups spinach
- 2 artichoke hearts
- 1 tsp cream cheese
- Grain salt

Preparation:

1. Cook the spinach with a little grain salt, drain and cool.
2. Chop the cucumbers and reserve
3. Chop the artichoke hearts into four, add them in a bowl with the spinach.
4. Add the cream cheese, seasoning and mixing everything.

Focaccia Bread With Garlic And Rosemary

Ingredients:

- 175 g (375 m) shredded mozzarella.
- 2 tbsp (30g) cream cheese.
- 1 tsp. white wine vinegar.
- 1 egg.
- 175 ml (100 g) ground almonds.
- ½ tsp of salt.
- ½ tsp garlic powder.
- 50 g butter at room temperature.
- 3 cloves garlic, finely chopped
- ½ teaspoon of sea salt
- ½ tsp fresh chopped rosemary

Preparation:

1. Preheat oven to 200 °C (400 °F)
2. Heat cream cheese and mozzarella cheese in a saucepan over medium heat (microwaves can also be used) and stir occasionally.
3. Add the rest of the ingredients and mix.
4. Flatten the dough to a round shape, no more than 20 cm above the baking paper.
5. Using a fork, make small holes, bake for 12 minutes or until golden brown, then remove and let cool.
6. Prepare a mixture with garlic, butter, salt and rosemary, spread on bread and place on a grill or grill

7.   Leave for 7 minutes

Mexican-Style Sausages

Ingredients:

- ½ cup chopped onion
- ½ tomato
- 2 turkey sausages
- Chili
- Grain salt

Preparation:

1.   Add onion in a pan over medium heat until translucent.
2.   Add the chili together with the tomato chopped in cubes, season with salt.
3.   Chop the sausages in slices and add the sauce, let cook and serve.

Lettuce Cubes With Prickly Pear Salad

Ingredients:

- Lettuce (4 firm leaves well washed)
- 2 prickly pears
- Grain salt
- ½ cup onion
- 1 tsp olive oil
- 1 tsp vinegar
- 1 tbsp. chopped coriander
- 1 small chili-tomato

Preparation:

1.   In a refractory add the prickly pears in cubes and leave them overnight with salt in grain (well covered).
2.   Next day drain and let dry

3. Cut the onion and tomato into cubes and add them to the nopales.

4. Add olive oil, chopped coriander, and vinegar.

5. Place the mixture on the lettuce

Prepared Olives

Ingredients:

- 1 lemon (juice)
- ¼ cup chopped onion
- 6 Kalamata olives, pitted and stuffed
- 2 tbsp soy sauce

Preparation:

1. Cook the onion in a frying pan until translucent.

2. Add the olives and sprinkle with the sauce and lemon.

3. Let cool and serve

Cauliflower Bits With Peanut Butter

Ingredients:

- 2 tbsp peanut butter
- coarse salt
- 1 tbsp olive oil
- 1 cauliflower

Preparation:

1. Preheat oven to 400°F (200°C)

2. Cut the cauliflower

3. On a tray with waxed paper, put the cauliflowers and add olive oil, season and bake until golden brown.

4. Remove from oven and spread peanut butter, bake for a couple more minutes.

5. Remove from oven, let cool and serve

Additionally, for those who need something fast due to their short time due to work or travel, there are adequate snacks to the keto diet, among the most prominent are:

- Packaged olives (green, black or assorted)
- Beef bar (shredded pork or chicken sriracha)
- Cooked bacon
- Salami snacks
- Pork cracklings
- Macadamia nuts
- Pili nuts
- Very dark chocolate

Chard Skewers With Ham And Cheese

Ingredients:
- 3 thin slices of cooked ham
- 3 thin slices of cheese
- 3 leaves of chard well cleaned
- 2 large tomatoes, well washed

Preparation:
Cook the chard for a maximum time of 2 minutes, take it out of the water and then let it cool until it can be manipulated. Then, place it on a tray or plate and put on it the slices of ham and cheese carefully to avoid breaking the chards and roll them up. We chop in rolls and we take out three portions to assemble the skewer placing in each end a cube of tomato, then to serve. This recipe of skewers is perfect to consume between meals as a salty snack, however for the one that prefers, it can be a recipe for a dinner rich in proteins.

Crackers Of Crunchy Seeds And Oats

Ingredients:

- 20 grams of poppy seeds
- 20 grams of linseed
- 25 grams of chia seeds
- 55 grams of sesame seed
- 55 grams of pumpkin seeds
- 20 grams of thin layers of oats
- ¼ of caraway seeds
- ¼ teaspoon of granulated garlic or a clove of grated garlic
- 250ml of water

Preparation:

Turn on the oven at 150°C, place all the ingredients in a container except for the water, mix them all very well, add the water stirring little by little until it integrates with all the ingredients, leave to rest well covered for 10 minutes. After the time has elapsed, check that the water has been absorbed by the seeds. Its consistency should be a sticky dough where not even a drop should be left, otherwise, add a little oatmeal or chia, mix and wait again.

Place in the tray greased paper and then flatten using a roller or a kitchen spatula, the mixture should not be more than 3 to 5mm thick, put in the oven for a time of 30 to 35 minutes. After that time, with the spatula, introduce underneath the mixture, trying to turn very carefully to prevent it from breaking (you can use board or large plate), bake again for 25 to 30 minutes more, be careful to avoid burning. Remove from the oven, wait for it to cool down, cut on a board and cut with a good knife into pieces.

Chapter 18:

Keto drinks

As well as the Keto diet offers us varieties in sweet tooths and snacks to be consumed without any remorse, it also provides us different drinks and smoothies that are allowed and are within the ketogenic standards. Here we show you the different options so that you can choose according to your preference:

Keto Smoothie Chocolate

Have a necessary quantity of zucchini, coconut milk, and lettuce at your disposal. Romana, chia seeds, spinach, cocoa powder, avocado, sweetener of Passion fruit and mix everything to obtain a rich and sweet drink.

Chia seeds with blueberries and coconut

- 1 cup cashew or almond milk
- 2 tbsp. coconut oil
- 2 tbsp. ground chia seeds
- Sweetener equivalent to 2 tablespoons of sugar
- 1 cup blueberries
- 1 cup Greek yogurt (can be substituted for coconut milk without milk)
- ½ cup coconut

Mix all ingredients

Smoothie For Breakfast

It is a rich cocktail ideal to start the day based on the following ingredients: Spinach, coconut milk, greens powder, whey protein, almonds, Brazil nuts, spinach, sweet potato starch, and psyllium seeds; optionally, you can add some almonds to give a greater nutty flavor, then mix all the ingredients together and you'll get a nutritious drink to start the day.

Green shake

You only need the necessary amount of lemon, cucumber, avocado, and kale, all this is mixed with water, then blended and ready, is a rich and healthy drink

Smoothie with almond milk

This drink apart from being rich and healthy provides nutrients needed to start the day, you will only need celery, cucumber, matcha, spinach, avocado, and almond milk, then mix all the ingredients and finally, we add the chia seeds and coconut oil

Chia shake

This drink provides us with fiber

Ingredients:

- 1 tbsp walnut butter
- 1 tablespoon of chia seeds (soaked in water for 10 minutes)
- ¼ cup coconut milk
- 1 avocado
- 2 tsp. cocoa beans (if you want to add more flavor)
- 1 tsp. cocoa powder
- 1 scoop of chocolate protein powder
- 1 tbsp coconut oil

Blend all the ingredients mixing uniformly. If it is too thick, you can add 1 cup of water. At the moment of serving you can decorate with cocoa beans and cinnamon.

Green milkshake (without dairy products)

It is called green milkshake because it is the predominant color, the ingredients to use are avocado, kiwi, fresh ginger, fresh parsley, raw cucumber, fresh pineapple, and lettuce. We blend all the ingredients with water and we sweeten with any sugar substitute that is to your liking and preference.

Smoothie with macadamia nut oil

To prepare this shake you only need to mix avocado, spinach, stevia, coconut milk, cream, macadamia nut oil, vanilla protein, and oil of avocado, if you don't want to add or you don't have avocado oil at your disposal it can be replaced by olive oil or peanut oil.

Milkshake of almonds and blueberries

What it is necessary to achieve this tasty and nutrient-rich drink is to combine sugar-free almond sugar, a small amount of blueberries preferably organic, almond butter (it must be raw) and MCT oil

Strawberry milkshake

To achieve an excellent blend and obtain this smoothie it is necessary:

- 1 cup of fresh strawberries
- 1 tsp vanilla extract
- 1 tbsp coconut oil (you can also use any other healthy oil)
- 450ml coconut milk, if not available can be replaced by a cup of Greek yogurt if you prefer a milkshake (add water if it's too thick).

Raspberry vanilla smoothie

Ingredients:

- ½ cup natural strawberries (can be frozen)
- ½ cup unsweetened coconut milk
- 2/3 cup water
- ½ vanilla tsp (extract)

Then mix all the ingredients in the blender

Beet Smoothie

Mix in the blender the following ingredients to enjoy a delicious smoothie.

- 1 tbsp coconut oil
- 1 tbsp whey protein
- 1 tsp powdered cinnamon
- 1 cup almond milk, coconut milk can also be used
- 1 tbsp powdered beet

Walnut Smoothie:

- 1 pinch of salt
- 1 tsp powdered cinnamon
- 1 tablespoon peanut butter or cashew butter
- 2 tbsp preferably ground flax seeds
- 2 tbsp peeled walnuts
- 1 cup almonds

Combine all ingredients and blend

Ginger Smoothie

- Ingredients for its preparation:
- 30g frozen spinach
- 2 tbsp lemon juice
- 150ml of water
- 2 tsp. fresh stuffed ginger
- 75ml coconut cream or coconut milk

Combine all ingredients, add tablespoons of lemon one at a time. one to achieve the desired taste, after serving the drink we add a little of grated ginger and sprinkle over it.

Ketogenic coffee with cinnamon

This drink is ideal for those cold days, to make it you will need the following ingredients:

- 1 tsp ground cinnamon

- 475ml of water
- 2 tbsp ground coffee
- 75ml whipping cream

We combine the coffee with the cinnamon. We add the water and make it like coffee is normally made. Beat the cream with the help of a mixer until you get a mixture to point of snow, we serve in a large cup the coffee, add the whipped cream over it and finally add the cinnamon.

Chai tea

It is a warm and aromatic drink perfect for cold and rainy days.

Ingredients:

- 475ml of water
- 75ml whipping cream
- 1 tbsp chai tea

Follow the instructions on the chai tea container (hot water and tea), in the microwave, heat the cream in a medium cup and add the tea.

Coffee with pumpkinspices

Ingredients:

- ½ Tbsp vanilla extract
- 1 tbsp (25g) erythritol
- 1 tsp. spice mix for pumpkin pie
- 60ml (60g) pumpkin puree
- 60ml decaffeinated espresso coffee can also be strong coffee
- 225ml hot, unsweetened almond milk

Preparation:

Add all the ingredients in a blender and blend until a soft mixture is obtained, try it and give it the taste according to your preference, finally serve it.

Eggnog

Ingredients:

- ¼ honey tsp
- 1 pinch of ground nutmeg
- 225ml whipping cream
- 1 orange, the zest, and the juice
- 4 tbsp. brandy or any dark liqueur
- ¼ Tbsp vanilla extract

Preperation:

1. Mix the honey, vanilla powder and beaten egg yolks until the mixture is smooth, add ¼ of orange. Then we add 4 tablespoons of juice of orange, with the liqueur, carefully mix the whipping cream and combine it in a bowl with the egg mixture.
2. Serve in glasses and take to the refrigerator for 15 minutes.
3. This helps to develop more flavor and consistency in the eggnog

Flavored water

The cold flavored water refreshes when we feel like something without the need of adding calories Ingredients:

- 1 liter of cold, freshwater
- Flavorings of your free choice that can be fresh mint, cucumber or raspberries
- 475ml of ice

Preparation

1- Add the cold water in a pitcher
2- Place the chosen flavor and take it to the refrigerator leaving it to rest for at least 30 minutes
3- Fresh mint, citrus fruits such as orange, lemon or berries can be added if desired
4- With only a few slices are enough to give a rich flavor

Cold coffee

To soothe the heat, this delicious iced drink is an excellent choice.

Ingredients:

- 60ml whipping cream
- 225ml of coffee
- Ice cubes
- Vanilla extract (optional)

Instructions

1- As usual prepare the coffee, but twice as usual and leave it to cool down.

2- In a large glass add the ice cubes, add the coffee and then the cream.

3- Serve

Coffee with ketogenic cream

Ingredients:

- 60ml whipping cream
- 180ml of coffee

Preparation:

1- Choose the coffee of your preference and prepare it as usual.

2- In a small pot add the cream and heat, stir gently until it becomes frothy

3- In a large cup, pour the hot cream, add the coffee and stir

4- Serve instantly accompanied by a handful of yummy walnuts.

Keto Cheesecake

Ingredients:

- 2 passion fruit
- 2 tablespoons ricotta cheese
- 1 sachet of stevia
- 1 glass almond milk
- ice to taste

Preparation:

Add all the ingredients in a blender, mix everything and you're done. This way we'll get a delicious drink.

Chapter 19: 7
Day Meal Plan:

The 7-day meal plan aims to give a general idea of how the ketogenic diet might work effectively, however it is important to remember that it may work differently in each body.

This plan is based on a diet high in fat, low in carbohydrates and moderate in protein on which we could base the first week of our keto diet, however, we can refer to previous chapters for more recipes.

Monday

Breakfast: 2 sausages rolled in turkey with feta cheese and green tea

Snack: keto chocolate cheesecake

Lunch: Chicken Salad

Snack: pork rinds

Dinner: steamed vegetables and salmon

Tuesday

Breakfast: Cheese and mushroom omelet

Snack: Coffee without sugar

Lunch: Mexican Chicken Tacos

Snack: squares of ham and cheese

Dinner: Shrimp brochettes with bacon and onion

Wednesday

Breakfast: 2 boiled eggs wrapped in bacon strips and avocado strips with green tea

Snack: Light gelatin

Lunch: Chicken breast stuffed with ham and cream cheese.

Snack: Celery sticks with guacamole

Dinner: chop suey

Thursday

Breakfast: Turkey sausage and blended protein with strawberries

Snack: 40 grams of peanuts

Lunch: Steamed broccoli with fish

Snack: Nuts

Dinner: Fish skewers with bell pepper

Friday

Breakfast: Keto waffles with egg, cheese, and bacon

Snack: Coffee

Lunch: Asian-style sauteed keto cabbage

snack: gelatine

dinner: ham and cheese rolls

Saturday

Breakfast: salmon and bell pepper omelet

Snack: Merey

Lunch: Keto Caprese Omelet

Snack: Keto Smoothie

Dinner: Beef wraps

Sunday

Breakfast: Low-carbohydrate banana waffles

Snack: keto chocolate cake

Lunch: Ketogenic Tex Mex Casserole

Snack: Coconut biscuits without oven

Dinner: Stuffed avocados with smoked salmon

Conclusion

Thank you for making it through to the end of Keto for women: The ultimate beginners guide to know your food needs, weight loss, diabetes prevention and boundless energy with high-fat ketogenic diet recipes, let's hope it was informative and able to provide you with all of the tools you need to achieve your goals whatever they may be.

Now that you made it to the end of the book, you may know some, not to say all, of the benefits that the keto diet will have in your body. Even though it may be really hard to get started into this feeding plan, it absolutely worth it. Do not give up, fight for what you want, learn what your body needs and give it to it.

Women are known for being brave, amazing fighters and really strong so, are you going to let some extra pounds turn you down? As you could read, this diet is not only made for losing weight, there are studies that prove that this diet helps people who suffer from diabetes, decreases the symptoms of POS, helps in menstruation problems, improves brain and many other organs of our body.

Please, remember that even if you understood everything that is written in this book, and you feel like you can go keto on your own, it really recommended to go with a nutritionist or a specialist in the area for what you are using keto diet for. For example, if you are using keto to control POS, visit first your gyno.

Finally, if you found this book useful in any way, a review on Amazon is always appreciated!

Keto Chaffle Cookbook

An Easy Guide to Make Delicious Chaffles with Low Carb Recipes to Lose Weight, Improve Your Health and Satisfy your soul. With Pictures!

By

Sofia Wilson

Introduction

Ketogenic refers to a low-carbohydrate diet. The aim is to eat more calories from fat and protein while eating fewer calories from carbohydrates. The carbohydrates that are easiest to digest, such as starch, pastries, soda, and white bread, are the first to go. When you consume fewer than 50 g of carbohydrates a day, your body easily runs out of energy. This normally takes three or four days. Then you'll begin to break down fat and protein for energy, potentially resulting in weight loss. Ketosis is the term for this state. It's crucial to remember that the ketogenic diet is a short-term diet designed to help you lose weight rather than change your lifestyle. A ketogenic diet is more often used to reduce weight, although it may also be used to treat medical problems such as epilepsy. It can even benefit those suffering from heart failure, some brain disorders, and even acne, although further study is required. Since the keto diet contains too much fat, adherents must ingest fat at every meal time. In a normal 2K-calorie diet, that would seem like 165 g of fat, 40 g of carbohydrates, and 75 g of protein. The exact ratio, on the other hand, is determined by your basic requirements. Nuts (walnuts, almonds), avocados, seeds, olive oil and tofu are among the healthier unsaturated fats allowed on the keto diet. However, oils (coconut, palm), butter, lard, and peanut butter all contain high amounts of saturated fats. Protein is an essential aspect of the keto diet, although it is also difficult to discern between protein items that are lean and protein products rich in fat(saturated), such as beef, bacon, and pork. What for fruits and vegetables? While fruits are generally rich in carbohydrates, unique fruits may be obtained in limited quantities (generally berries) Leafy greens (like kale, chard, Swiss chard, and spinach), broccoli, cauliflower, asparagus, tomatoes, brussels sprouts, bell peppers, garlic, cucumbers, mushrooms, summer squashes, as well as celery are also rich in carbohydrates. One cup of sliced broccoli includes about six carbohydrates. At the same time, there are several possible keto hazards, such as liver deficiency, liver complications, constipation, kidney disorders, and so on. As a result, we can also keep our Keto diet portions in check.

Understanding The Ketogenic Diet

This chapter delves into the Ketogenic diet in depth. The chapter further discusses which foods to consume on the Keto diet and which foods to stop while on this diet. The Keto diet is often explained in-depth, including how it functions and what health advantages it provides.

The ketogenic diet (or keto diet) is a high-fat, low-carbohydrate diet with various health benefits. Evidently, more than 20 studies suggest that this form of diet will help you lose weight and boost your wellbeing. Diabetes patients, epilepsy patients, patients suffering from Alzheimer's disease, as well as cancer can all benefit from ketogenic diets.

1.1 What is Keto?

The ketogenic diet is a very low carbohydrate, high-fat diet that has a lot in common with the Atkins diet and other low-carb diets. It necessitates a significant reduction of carbohydrate consumption and a replacement with fat. This reduction of carbohydrates puts the body into a metabolic condition known as ketosis. As this occurs, the body's energy production of fat-burning skyrockets. In addition, it converts fat into ketones in the liver, which will supply energy to the brain. Ketogenic diets can result in substantial reductions in insulin as well as blood sugar levels. This, along with the increased ketones, has numerous health benefits.

Ketogenic Diets Come in Many Forms

There are a few variations of the ketogenic diet, including:

The traditional ketogenic diet consists of a diet that is low in carbs, mild in protein, and strong in fats. It usually has a 75 percent fat content, a 5% carbohydrate content, and a 20% protein content.

The cyclic ketogenic diet entails high-carb reefed cycles, such as five ketogenic days accompanied by two days of high carbohydrate use.

A ketogenic diet with particular goals: The diet requires carbs to be inserted in between exercises.

Protein-rich ketogenic diet: This is comparable to a normal keto diet, but it contains extra protein. Usually, the ratio is 60 percent fat, 5% sugars, and 35 percent protein.

However, only normal and protein-rich ketogenic diets have been extensively studied. More complex keto diets, such as targeted or cyclic keto, are mainly utilized by bodybuilders and athletes.

Ketogenic Diet Health Benefits

In fact, the keto diet first gained popularity as a means of treating neurological conditions, such as epilepsy. Following that, research has shown that diet can help with a broad variety of health issues:

Heart disease: The keto diet has been found to decrease risk factors such as body fat, blood sugar, HDL cholesterol and blood pressure.

Alzheimer's disease: The ketogenic diet can ease Alzheimer's symptoms while still delaying the disease's progression.

Epilepsy: Research has demonstrated that a ketogenic diet can significantly reduce seizures in children with epileptic seizures.

Cancer: The diet is actually being used to control a number of diseases and to delay tumor development.

Acne: Lower insulin levels, as well as less sugar or fried food diets, will aid acne recovery.

Parkinson's disease: According to one report, diet can help relieve the effects of Parkinson's disease.

Brain injuries: One study found that the diet would also increase concussions and improve recovery after a brain injury.

Polycystic ovary syndrome: A ketogenic diet may help lower insulin levels and can be helpful in the treatment of polycystic ovary syndrome.

What foods can you consume on a ketogenic diet?

The majority of your meals will revolve around the following foods:

- Salmon, mackerel and tuna are representations of fatty fish.
- Look for pastured eggs, whole eggs, or omega-3 eggs.
- Seek for grass-fed butter plus cream wherever possible.
- Red meat, ham, sausage, turkey, bacon, chicken and steak are all examples of meat.
- Non-processed cheese (goat, cheddar, mozzarella, blue, or cream).
- Flax seeds, walnuts, almonds, pumpkin seeds, chia seeds and other nuts and beans
- Avocado oil, olive oil and coconut oil are the other safe oils.
- Salt, spices and pepper, as well as a variety of herbs, may be used as condiments.
- Avocados: entire avocados or guacamole made freshly.
- Low-carb vegetables including greens, tomatoes, onions, peppers and other related veggies.

Foods to avoid on a ketogenic diet include:

Carbohydrate-rich diets can be avoided as much as possible.

The following is a selection of items that must be eliminated or reduced on a ketogenic diet:

- Sugary drink, ice cream, soda, smoothies, cake, candy and other sugary items
- Wheat, pasta, cereals, rice, and other wheat-based products are examples of starches or grains.
- Sweet potatoes, parsnips, parsnips, potatoes, carrots and other tubers & root vegetables
- Reduced-calorie or low-fat foods are extremely processed and abundant in carbohydrates.
- Fruit: All fruits, with the exception of tiny bits of berries like strawberries.
- Chickpeas, lentils, peas, kidney beans, and other legumes or beans
- Some sauces/condiments: They are also high in unhealthy fat and sugar.

- Unhealthy fats: Limit the intake to mayonnaise, processed vegetable oils, and other processed fats.
- Alcohol: Because of their carb content, certain alcoholic beverages will shake you out of ketosis.
- Dietary ingredients that are sugar-free: Alcohols, which are often rich in sugar, may influence ketone levels in certain situations. These objects seem to have passed through a lot of refining as well.

1.2 What is the Keto diet, and how does it work?

The "ketogenic" keto diet consists of consuming a moderate level of protein, a heavy amount of fat, and relatively little carbohydrates; also, the fruit is forbidden. As for every diet fad, the advantages to adherents include improved vitality, weight reduction, and mental clarity. Is the ketogenic diet, though, what it's cracked up to be?

Dietitians and nutritionists are quiet on the topic. Low-carb diets like keto appear to assist with weight loss in the short term, but they are no more successful than any other self-help or conventional diet. They still don't seem to be enhancing athletic results.

The ketogenic diet was created to treat epilepsy instead of losing weight. In the 1920s, physicians found that holding people on low-carb diets induced their bodies to use fat as the predominant fuel source rather than glucose. When only fat is available for the body to combust or burn, the body converts fats to fatty acids, which are then converted to ketones, which can be used and taken up to power the body's cells.

Currently, feeding the body exclusively ketones prevents epilepsy for unclear causes. However, with the advent of anti-seizure medicines, few patients with epilepsy rely on ketogenic diets anymore, while certain people who may not respond to medications may benefit. Low carb diets like the Atkins diet, which gained popularity in the early 2000s, also spawned keto diets for weight loss. In comparison, all groups of meatier-meal diets restrict carbohydrates. This diet does not have a set structure, although most routines provide for fewer than fifty grams of carbs per day.

A keto diet causes the body to enter a state known as ketosis, in which the body's cells become completely reliant on ketones for nutrition. It's not exactly clear that this leads to weight loss, but ketosis decreases appetite and can affect hunger-controlling hormones, including insulin. As a consequence, proteins and fats can keep humans fuller longer than sugars, resulting in lower net calorie intake.

In one head-to-head comparison, researchers looked at 48 separate diet trials in which subjects were randomly allocated to one of the well-known diets. Low-carb diets like South Beach, Atkins, and Zone, as well as low-fat diets like Ornish diets and portion restriction diets like Weight Watchers and Jenny Craig, were among the options.

Every diet resulted in greater weight loss than almost no diet after six months, according to the results. Low-carb and low-fat dieters lost almost equal amounts of weight as compared to non-dieters, with low-carb dieters losing 19 pounds on average versus low-fat dieters dropping 17.6 pounds (7.99 kilograms). At 12 months, both diet styles displayed symptoms of dropping off, with low-fat and low-carb dieters being 16 pounds (7.27 kg) smaller on average than non-dieters.

There were few differences in weight reduction within the diets of designated people. This is in line with the practice of recommending every diet that an individual practice in order to lose weight.

Another study of well-known diets discovered the Atkins diet, which results in greater weight loss than merely teaching people about portion control. Nevertheless, several of the scientific researched about this low-carb diet featured licensed dietitians assisting respondents in making food decisions, rather than the self-directed approach used by most people. This has been seen in other diet studies, according to the researchers, and the tests' results seem to be more positive in the real world than the weight loss.

Finally, a simple comparison between low-carb versus low-fat dieting revealed that there was a statistically significant difference in the amount of weight lost over a year. Low-carbohydrate dieters dropped an average of 13 pounds (6 kg), compared to 11.7 pounds for low-fat dieters (5.3 kg).

Ketogenic diets may help us lose weight, but they are no more successful than other diet methods. Since carbohydrate reserves in the body comprise water molecules, the bulk of the weight lost during the early stages of a ketogenic diet is water weight. This gives the scale an exciting amount at first, but weight reduction slows down with time.

What are the keto effects, and how can they help?

The advantages of a keto diet are close to that of other high-fat, low-carb diets, but it tends to be more successful than centrist low-carb diets. Keto is a low-carb, high-fat diet that maximizes health benefits. However, it will slightly raise the likelihood of complications.

Aid in weight loss

Weight reduction can be improved by converting the body into a fat-burning device. Insulin levels – the hormone that retains fat – are falling rapidly, suggesting that fat burning has risen dramatically. This seems to make it much easier to lose bodyweight without going hungry.

More than thirty high-quality observational studies show that low-carb and keto diets are more effective than other diets at losing weight.

Reverse type 2 diabetes by regulating blood sugar

A ketogenic diet has been shown in research to be successful in the treatment of type 2 diabetes, with total disease reversal occurring in certain instances. It makes perfect sense since keto removes the need for therapy, lowers blood sugar levels, and eliminates the potential negative consequences of high insulin levels.

Since a keto diet will reverse type 2 diabetes, it is likely to be helpful in preventing and reversing pre-diabetes. Keep in mind that "reversal" in this context refers to changing the disease, improving glucose tolerance, and reducing the need for care. It may be so drastically altered that after therapy, blood pressure returns to normal with time. In this context, reversal refers to progressing or deteriorating in the reverse direction of the condition. Changes in your lifestyle, on the other side, just succeed if you bring them into effect. If a person returns to the way of life he or she has before diabetes type 2 appeared and advanced, it is possible that success would return with time.

Improve your mental and physical performance:

Some people use ketogenic diets to boost their mental performance. It's also normal for people to feel more energized while they're in ketosis.

They don't need nutritional carbs for the brain on keto. It runs on ketones 24 hours a day, seven days a week, with a small amount of glucose synthesized in the liver. Carbohydrates are not necessary for the diet. As a result, ketosis leads to a steady flow of food (ketones) to the brain, avoiding significant blood sugar spikes. This will also assist with improved focus and attention, as well as clearing brain fog and improving mental awareness.

Epilepsy Treatment

The keto diet has been used to manage epilepsy since the 19th and 20th centuries and has proved to be effective. It has historically been used mainly for adolescents, although in recent years, it has also proved to be useful to adults. Or, used in conjunction with a keto diet, certain people with epilepsy might be able to take less to no anti-epileptic drugs while being seizure-free. This may help to reduce the drug's adverse effects while still improving cognitive capacity.

Keto Chaffle Recipes

1 Oreo Chaffles

(Ready in about 23 minutes | Serving 2 | Difficulty: Easy)

Per serving: Kcal 1381, Fat: 146g, Net Carbs: 14g, Protein: 17g

Ingredients

- 1/2 cup of Sugar-Free Chocolate Chips
- 1 tsp of Vanilla extract
- 3 Eggs
- 1/2 cup of butter
- 1/4 cup of sweetener

Cheese Frosting

- 4 ounces of Cream Cheese
- 4 ounces of butter
- 1/2 cup of Powdered Swerve
- 1 tsp of Vanilla extract
- 1/4 cup of Whipping Cream

Instructions

Melt chocolate and butter in a bowl in the microwave for around 1 minute. Stir to remove clumps. Mix vanilla, egg and sweetener in a bowl. Pour a quarter of the mixture into the waffle maker and cook for around 8 minutes. Mix frosting ingredients in the food processor's bowl in the meantime and make a smooth mixture. Spread frosting among two chaffles.

2 Strawberry Chaffles

(Ready in about 35 minutes | Serving 8 | Difficulty: Moderate)

Per serving: Kcal 189, Fat: 14.3g, Net Carbs: 5.2g, Protein: 10g

Ingredients

- 3 oz of cream cheese
- 1 cup of whipped cream
- 2 beaten eggs
- 2 cups shredded mozzarella cheese
- 1/2 cup of almond flour
- 2 tsp of baking powder
- 3 tbsp of sweetener
- 8 strawberries
- 1 tbsp of sweetener

Instructions

Add mozzarella and cream cheese to a bowl and microwave for around 1 minute. Beat eggs and mix with baking powder, 3 tbsp sweetener and almond flour. Mix it with cheese and add to 2 diced strawberries. Place in the fridge for around 20 minutes. Dice the rest of the strawberries and add tbsp sweetener. Warm waffle iron and add the quarter mixture from the fridge to the center of the iron. Cook for around 7 minutes.

3 Chocolate Chaffle

(Ready in about 18 minutes | Serving 2 | Difficulty: Easy)

Per serving: Kcal 672, Fat: 70g, Net Carbs: 11g, Protein: 13g

Ingredients

- 1/2 cup of Chocolate Chips
- 1/4 cup of sweetener
- 3 Eggs
- 1/2 cup of butter
- 1 tsp of Vanilla extract

Instructions

Melt chocolate and butter in a bowl in the microwave for around 1 minute. Stir and remove clumps. Blend sweetener, vanilla and eggs in a bowl. Add chocolate and butter and whisk. Pour the quarter amount of mixture into a waffle maker. Cook for around 8 minutes.

4 Pumpkin Chaffles

(Ready in about 7 minutes | Serving 1 | Difficulty: Easy)

Per serving: Kcal 250, Fat: 15g, Net Carbs: 5g, Protein: 23g

Ingredients

- 1/2 cup mozzarella cheese shredded
- 1 1/2tbsp of pumpkin purée
- 1 beaten egg
- 1/2tsp of Swerve confectioners
- 1/4tsp of Pumpkin Pie Spice
- 1/2tsp of vanilla extract
- ⅛ tsp of maple extract

Instructions

Mix all the ingredients except mozzarella cheese in a bowl and mix. Add cheese and whisk. Spray waffle using cooking spray. Place half amount of batter in the center of the waffle maker. Cook for around 6 minutes. Repeat with the remaining batter.

5 Basic Chaffle

(Ready in about 8 minutes | Serving 2 | Difficulty: Easy)

Per serving: Kcal 208, Fat: 16g, Net Carbs: 4g, Protein: 11g

Ingredients

- 1 Big Egg
- 2 tbsp of Almond Flour
- 1/2 cup shredded Mozzarella cheese

Instructions

Preheat waffle iron for around 5 minutes. Microwave cheese for around 30 seconds. Add the rest of the ingredients and mix. Pour mixture that covers the surface of the waffle maker. Cook for around 4 minutes. Take out and place on a plate and repeat with the rest of the batter.

6 Garlic Chaffles

(Ready in about 8 minutes | Serving 2 | Difficulty: Easy)

Per serving: Kcal 208, Fat: 16g, Net Carbs: 4g, Protein: 11g

Ingredients

- 1/3 cup Parmesan cheese Grated
- 1/2 cup shredded Mozzarella cheese
- 1 Big Egg
- 1/2 tsp of Italian seasoning
- 1 minced Garlic clove

Instructions

Preheat waffle iron for around 5 minutes. Microwave cream cheese for around 30 seconds. Add the rest of the ingredients except the toppings. Pour mixture that covers the surface of the waffle maker. Cook for around 4 minutes. Take out and place on a plate and repeat with the rest of the batter.

© BudgetMomma.com

7 Cinnamon Chaffles

(Ready in about 8 minutes | Serving 2 | Difficulty: Easy)

Per serving: Kcal 208, Fat: 16g, Net Carbs: 4g, Protein: 11g

Ingredients

- 3/4 cup shredded Mozzarella cheese
- 1 Big Egg
- 2 tbsp of Almond Flour
- 2 tbsp of besti erythritol
- 1/2 tbsp melted butter
- 1/2 tsp of cinnamon
- 1 tbsp melted butter
- 1/2 tsp of vanilla extract
- 3/4 tsp of cinnamon
- 1/4 cup of besti erythritol

Instructions

Preheat waffle iron for around 5 minutes. Microwave cream cheese for around 30 seconds. Add the rest of the ingredients except the toppings. Pour mixture that covers the surface of the waffle maker. Cook for around 4 minutes. Take out and place on a plate and repeat with the rest of the batter. To prepare churro chaffles, mix cinnamon and erythritol for topping. Brush chaffles using butter after they are cooked and sprinkle with topping.

8 Cheese Chaffles

(Ready in about 8 minutes | Serving 2 | Difficulty: Easy)

Per serving: Kcal 208, Fat: 16g, Net Carbs: 4g, Protein: 11g

Ingredients

- 1 Egg
- 1/2 oz of Cream cheese
- 1/2 cup shredded Mozzarella cheese
- 2 1/2 tbsp of Besti Erythritol
- 2 tbsp of pumpkin puree
- 1/2 tbsp of Pumpkin pie spice
- 3 tsp of Coconut Flour

Instructions

Preheat waffle iron for around 5 minutes. Microwave cream cheese for around 30 seconds. Add the rest of the ingredients except the toppings. Pour mixture that covers the surface of the waffle maker. Cook for around 4 minutes. Take out and place on a plate and repeat with the rest of the batter.

9 Spicy Chaffles

(Ready in about 8 minutes | Serving 2 | Difficulty: Easy)

Per serving: Kcal 208, Fat: 16g, Net Carbs: 4g, Protein: 11g

Ingredients

- 1 Egg
- 1 oz of Cream cheese
- 1 cup shredded Cheddar cheese
- 1/2 tbsp of Jalapenos
- 2 tbsp of Bacon bits

Instructions

Preheat waffle iron for around 5 minutes. Microwave cream cheese for around 30 seconds. Add the rest of the ingredients except the toppings. Pour mixture that covers the surface of the waffle maker. Cook for around 4 minutes. Take out and place on a plate and repeat with the rest of the batter.

10 Double Chocolate Chaffles

(Ready in about 5 minutes | Serving 1 | Difficulty: Easy)

Per serving: Kcal 197, Fat: 23.3g, Net Carbs: 11.3g, Protein: 24.3g

Ingredients

- 1 egg
- 1 tbsp of granulated sweetener
- 1/2 cup grated mozzarella
- 1 tsp of vanilla
- 1 tbsp of chocolate chips
- 2 tbsp of almond meal/flour
- 1 tsp of heavy cream
- 2 tbsp unsweetened cocoa powder

Instructions

Add all the ingredients to a bowl and mix. Preheat the waffle maker. Spray with oil and pour half amount of batter into the maker. Cook for around 4 minutes. Sprinkle with toppings and enjoy.

11 Vanilla Chaffles

(Ready in about 10 minutes | Serving 1 | Difficulty: Easy)

Per serving: Kcal 184, Fat: 20.1g, Net Carbs: 5.4g, Protein: 22.2g

Ingredients

- 1/2 cup of grated mozzarella
- 1 tbsp of granulated sweetener
- 1 eggs
- 1 tsp of vanilla extract
- 1 tbsp of chocolate chips
- 2 tbsp of almond flour

Instructions

Combine all the ingredients in a bowl. Preheat the waffle maker and spray it using oil once it is hot. Pour half amount of batter in the maker and cook for around 4 minutes. Remove and do the same with the rest of the batter. Top and enjoy.

12 Lemon Curd Chaffle

(Ready in about 50 minutes | Serving 3 | Difficulty: Hard)

Per serving: Kcal 302, Fat: 24g, Net Carbs: 6g, Protein: 15g

Ingredients

- 3 eggs
- one batch of lemon curd
- 4 ounces softened cream cheese
- 1 tsp of vanilla extract
- 1 tbsp sweetener low carb
- 3/4 cup shredded mozzarella cheese
- 1 tsp of baking powder
- 3 tbsp of coconut flour
- 1/3 tsp of salt

Instructions

Prepare lemon curd according to package instructions. Heat the maker and spray oil. Mix baking powder, salt and coconut flour in a bowl. Add the rest of the ingredients to another bowl and beat using a hand blender. Mix the two bowls mixture and pour in the maker. Cook for around 5 minutes. Top using lemon curd.

13 Glazed Donut

(Ready in about 15 minutes | Serving 3 | Difficulty: Easy)

Per serving: Kcal 246, Fat: 17g, Net Carbs: 2g, Protein: 14g

Ingredients

For chaffles

- 1/2 cup shredded cheese Mozzarella
- 2 tbsp of whey protein
- 1 ounce of Cream Cheese
- 2 tbsp of Swerve confectioners
- 1/2tsp of Vanilla extract
- 1/2tsp of Baking powder
- 1 Egg

For glaze

- 1/2tsp of Vanilla extract
- 3-4 tbsp of Swerve confectioners
- 2 tbsp of whipping cream

Instructions

Preheat the waffle maker. Add cream cheese and mozzarella in a bowl and microwave for around 30 seconds. Add 2 tbsp sweetener, whey protein and baking powder and mix. Add dough to a bowl and break an egg into it and add vanilla. Stir to form a smooth mixture. Add batter to the waffle maker and cook for around 5 minutes. Beat glaze ingredients in a bowl and top chaffles with it.

14 Nut-Free Chaffles

(Ready in about 30 minutes | Serving 3 | Difficulty: Easy)

Per serving: Kcal 195, Fat: 15.1g, Net Carbs: 31.5g, Protein: 8.5g

Ingredients

Batter

- 1/2 cup shredded cheese mozzarella
- 1/4 tsp of vanilla extract
- 2 tbsp of SunButter
- 2 tbsp of fruit sweetener
- 1 egg
- 2 tsp of cinnamon
- 1 tbsp of coconut flour
- ⅛ tsp of baking powder

Frosting

- 1 tbsp of cream cheese
- 1/4 cup of fruit sweetener
- 3/4 tbsp of butter, melted
- 1 tbsp of coconut milk unsweetened
- 1/4 tsp of vanilla extract

Coating

- 1 tsp of fruit sweetener
- 1 tsp of cinnamon

Instructions

Preheat the waffle iron. Mix batter ingredients in a bowl and place aside. Mix frosting ingredients except for coconut milk in a bowl and whisk until smooth. Add coconut milk and mix again. Place aside. Coat iron with cooking spray and add batter. Cook for around 4 minutes. Sprinkle with sweetener and cinnamon.

15 Chicken Chaffle

(Ready in about 19 minutes | Serving 2 | Difficulty: Easy)

Per serving: Kcal 675, Fat: 52g, Net Carbs: 8g, Protein: 44g

Ingredients

- 1/4 cup of almond flour
- 1/4 cup crumbled feta cheese
- 2 eggs
- 1 tsp of baking powder
- 1/2 cup shredded chicken
- 1/4 cup of Hot Sauce
- 1/4 cup shredded mozzarella cheese
- 3/4 cup shredded cheddar cheese
- 1/4 cup diced celery

Instructions

Mix almond flour and baking powder in a bowl. Preheat iron and spray using cooking spray. Beat eggs in a bowl and add hot sauce. Combine thoroughly and pour flour mixture. Combine and add grated cheeses. Fold in chicken. Pour in the maker and cook for around 4 minutes. Top with celery and feta.

16 Chaffle Sandwich

(Ready in about 13 minutes | Serving 1 | Difficulty: Easy)

Per serving: Kcal 238, Fat: 18g, Net Carbs: 2g, Protein: 17g

Ingredients

For chaffles

- 1/2 cup shredded Cheddar cheese
- 1 egg

For sandwich

- 1 tbsp of mayonnaise
- 2 slices of tomato
- 2 strips of bacon
- 3 pieces of lettuce

Instructions

Preheat the maker and mix cheese and egg in a bowl. Pour batter into the maker and cook for around 4 minutes. Do it in 2 batches. Cook bacon in pan paced on the moderate flame until it gets crispy. Drain using paper towels and form a sandwich using tomato, mayonnaise and lettuce.

17 Sausage Gravy Chaffle

(Ready in about 15 minutes | Serving 2 | Difficulty: Easy)

Per serving: Kcal 212, Fat: 17g, Net Carbs: 3g, Protein: 11g

Ingredients

For Chaffle

- 1/2 cup grated mozzarella cheese
- 1 egg
- 1 tsp of coconut flour
- 1/4 tsp of baking powder
- 1 tsp of water
- Salt

For Gravy

- 3 tbsp of chicken broth
- 1/4 cup browned breakfast sausage
- 2 tbsp of whipping cream
- dash of garlic powder
- 2 tsp softened cream cheese
- pepper

Instructions

Preheat the maker and coat using cooking spray. Add all ingredients to a bowl and mix. Pour half amount to mixture into the maker and cook for around 4 minutes. Repeat with the remaining batter and enjoy. Prepare breakfast sausage and add in the pan with remaining ingredients and boil. Reduce flame and cook for around 7 minutes to thicken it. Add pepper and salt and spoon gravy on top of chaffles.

18 Eggs Benedict

(Ready in about 30 minutes | Serving 2 | Difficulty: Easy)

Per serving: Kcal 844, Fat: 78g, Net Carbs: 5g, Protein: 32g

Ingredients
For Chaffles
- 1/2 cup of mozzarella cheese
- 2 tbsp of almond flour
- 2 whites of eggs
- 1 tbsp of sour cream

For Hollandaise
- 2 tbsp of lemon juice
- 4 yolks of eggs
- 1/2 cup of salted butter

For Eggs
- 1 tbsp of white vinegar
- 3 ounces of deli ham
- 2 eggs

Instructions

Whisk eggs in a bowl and with the rest of the ingredients and blend. Preheat the waffle maker. Spray using cooking spray and add half the mixture. Cook for around 7 minutes. Make hollandaise sauce by forming a double broiler. Boil water and warm butter in the microwave. Add egg to bowl of the boiler. Boil and add hot butter while the pot is carried to a boil. Cook until egg thickens and take out of the bowl. Drizzle lemon juice and place aside. Warm chaffle using toaster and top with ham slices, 2 tbsp hollandaise sauce and one egg.

19 Garlic Chaffle

(Ready in about 10 minutes | Serving 8 | Difficulty: Easy)

Per serving: Kcal 74, Fat: 6.5g, Net Carbs: 0.9g, Protein: 3.4g

Ingredients

- 1 egg
- 2 tbsp of almond flour
- 1/2 cup grated mozzarella cheese
- 1/2tsp of garlic powder
- 1/2tsp of salt
- 1/2tsp of oregano

Topping

- 1/2tsp of garlic powder
- 2 tbsp softened butter
- 1/4 cup grated mozzarella cheese

Instructions

Preheat the maker and oil it. Mix ingredients except topping ingredients. Pour into the maker and cook for around 5 minutes. Mix garlic powder and butter and pour over waffle. Sprinkle with mozzarella and cook for around 3 minutes.

© MidgetMomma.com

20 Taco Chaffle

(Ready in about 13 minutes | Serving 1 | Difficulty: Easy)

Per serving: Kcal 258, Fat: 19g, Net Carbs: 4g, Protein: 18g

Ingredients

- 1/4 cup shredded jack cheese
- 1 white of egg
- 1/4 cup shredded cheddar cheese
- 1 tsp of coconut flour
- 3/4 tsp of water
- 1/4 tsp of baking powder
- pinch of salt
- 1/8 tsp of chili powder

Instructions

Preheat the maker and oil it. Combine everything in a bowl and spoon half amount of mixture in the maker. Cook for around 4 minutes. Remove the chaffle shell and place it aside. Repeat with the remaining batter. Turn the pan and position shells of the chaffle among cups to make a shell of taco.

21 Pizza Chaffle

(Ready in about 8 minutes | Serving 2 | Difficulty: Easy)

Per serving: Kcal 76, Fat: 4.3g, Net Carbs: 4.1g, Protein: 5.5g

Ingredients

- 1 egg
- Pinch of Italian seasoning
- 1/2 cup shredded mozzarella cheese
- 1 tbsp of pizza sauce

Instructions

Preheat the maker. Whisk eggs in a bowl and add seasonings. Mix shredded cheese in a bowl. Add half amount of mixture to the maker and cook for around 4 minutes. Repeat with the rest of the batter and with 1 tbsp pizza sauce and pepperoni.

22 Parmesan Chaffles

(Ready in about 6 minutes | Serving 1 | Difficulty: Easy)

Per serving: Kcal 352, Fat: 24g, Net Carbs: 2g, Protein: 14g

Ingredients

- 1 beaten egg
- 1/2 cup of mozzarella cheese shredded
- 1/4 cup of Parmesan cheese grated
- 1/4tsp of garlic powder
- 1 tsp of Italian seasoning

Instructions

Preheat the waffle maker. Add all the ingredients except mozzarella and parmesan cheese in a bowl and mix. Mix the cheese in a bowl and spray waffle sung cooking spray. Pour half amount of mixture in the maker and cook for around 5 minutes. Top using parmesan and enjoy.

CHICKEN PARMESAN Chaffle

23 Italian Chaffle

(Ready in about 6 minutes | Serving 1 | Difficulty: Easy)

Per serving: Kcal 352, Fat: 24g, Net Carbs: 2g, Protein: 14g

Ingredients

- 1 beaten egg
- 1/2 cup of mozzarella cheese shredded
- 1/4 cup of Parmesan cheese grated
- 1/4tsp of garlic powder
- 1 tsp of Italian seasoning

Instructions

Preheat the waffle maker. Add all the ingredients except mozzarella and parmesan cheese in a bowl and mix. Mix the cheese in a bowl and spray waffle sung cooking spray. Pour half amount of mixture in the maker and cook for around 5 minutes. Top using parmesan and add lettuce, cold cuts, tomato.

24 Chaffle Breadsticks

(Ready in about 6 minutes | Serving 1 | Difficulty: Easy)

Per serving: Kcal 352, Fat: 24g, Net Carbs: 2g, Protein: 14g

Ingredients

- 1 beaten egg
- 1/2 cup of mozzarella cheese shredded
- Marinara sauce
- 1/4 cup of Parmesan cheese grated
- 1/4tsp of garlic powder
- 1 tsp of Italian seasoning

Instructions

Preheat the waffle maker. Add all the ingredients except mozzarella and parmesan cheese in a bowl and mix. Mix the cheese in a bowl and spray waffle sung cooking spray. Pour half amount of mixture in the maker and cook for around 5 minutes. Top using parmesan and dice into 4 sticks and enjoy with Marinara Sauce.

25 Chaffle Bruschetta

(Ready in about 6 minutes | Serving 1 | Difficulty: Easy)

Per serving: Kcal 352, Fat: 24g, Net Carbs: 2g, Protein: 14g

Ingredients

- 1 beaten egg
- 1/2 cup of mozzarella cheese shredded
- 1/4 cup of Parmesan cheese grated
- Basil
- Olive oil
- 1/4tsp of garlic powder
- 1 tsp of Italian seasoning

Instructions

Preheat the waffle maker. Add all the ingredients except mozzarella and parmesan cheese in a bowl and mix. Mix the cheese in a bowl and spray waffle sung cooking spray. Pour half amount of mixture in the maker and cook for around 5 minutes. Top using parmesan and mix 4 chopped cherry tomatoes, ½ tsp chopped fresh basil, drop of olive oil and salt. Add on chaffle.

26 Cauliflower Chaffles

(Ready in about 9 minutes | Serving 2 | Difficulty: Easy)

Per serving: Kcal 246, Fat: 16g, Net Carbs: 7g, Protein: 20g

Ingredients

- 1/4 tsp of Garlic Powder
- 1 cup of riced cauliflower
- 1/4 tsp of Ground Black Pepper
- 1/4 tsp of Kosher Salt
- 1/2 tsp of Italian seasoning
- 1 Eggs
- 1/2 cup of mozzarella cheese shredded
- 1/2 cup of parmesan cheese shredded

Instructions

Blend all ingredients except the cauliflower mixture and parmesan cheese in a blender and sprinkle half parmesan in the maker. Pour mixture in maker and top with cauliflower mixture and rest of parmesan. Cook for around 5 minutes.

27 Zucchini Chaffles

(Ready in about 15 minutes | Serving 2 | Difficulty: Easy)

Per serving: Kcal 194, Fat: 13g, Net Carbs: 4g, Protein: 16g

Ingredients

- 1 beaten Egg
- 1/2 tsp Black Pepper Ground
- 1 cup grated Zucchini
- 1/2 cup of parmesan cheese shredded
- 1 tsp chopped Dried Basil
- 1/4 cup of mozzarella cheese shredded
- 3/4 tsp divided Kosher Salt

Instructions

Sprinkle 1/4 tsp salt on zucchini. Beat egg in a bowl and add mozzarella, zucchini, 1/2 tsp salt, basil and pepper. Sprinkle 2 tbsp parmesan on iron and spread a quarter of zucchini mixture on the maker. Top using 2 tbsp parmesan and cook for around 8 minutes. Repeat with the rest of the mixture.

28 Peanut Chaffles

(Ready in about 6 minutes | Serving 2 | Difficulty: Easy)

Per serving: Kcal 264, Fat: 21.6g, Net Carbs: 7.25g, Protein: 9.45g

Ingredients

Chaffle

- 1 Egg
- 1/4 tsp of Baking Powder
- 1 tbsp of Unsweetened Cocoa
- 1 tbsp of Heavy Cream
- 1 tbsp of Powdered Sweetener
- 1/2 tsp of Vanilla Extract
- 1 tsp of Coconut Flour
- 1/2 tsp of Batter Flavor

Butter Filling

- 2 tsp of Powdered Sweetener
- 3 tbsp of Peanut Butter
- 2 tbsp of Heavy Cream

InstructionsPreheat the maker. Combine ingredients of chaffle in a bowl and pour half amount of mixture in maker. Cook for around 5 minutes. Repeat with the rest of the mixture. Blend butter ingredients and spread over chaffles.

29 Easy Chaffle Recipe

(Ready in about 10 minutes | Serving 2| Difficulty: Easy)

Ingredients

Simple Chaffles

Per serving: Kcal 152, Fat: 8g, Net Carbs: 1g, Protein: 9g

- 1 Egg
- 1/2 Cup of Shredded Cheese Mozarella

Instructions

Add all ingredients to a bowl and whisk to combine. Coat waffle maker using cooking spray and pour half amount of batter into the maker. Cook for around 5 minutes and repeat with the rest of the batter.

30 Savory Chaffles

Per serving: Kcal 215, Fat: 16.5g, Net Carbs: 2g, Protein: 12g

- 1 Egg
- 1/2 Cup Shredded Cheese Mozarella
- 1/16 Tsp of Xanthan Gum
- 1/4 Cup of Almond Flour

Instructions

Add all ingredients to a bowl and whisk to combine. Coat waffle maker using cooking spray and pour half amount of batter into the maker. Cook for around 5 minutes and repeat with the rest of the batter.

31 Sweet Chaffles

Per serving: Kcal 192, Fat: 15gg, Net Carbs: 1.55g, Protein: 15g

- 1 Egg
- 1/2 Cup of Shredded Cheese Mozzarella
- 1/4 Cup of Almond Flour
- 1/16 Tsp of Xanthan Gum
- 2 Tbsp of Confectioners Swerve

Instructions

Add all ingredients to a bowl and whisk to combine. Coat waffle maker using cooking spray and pour half amount of batter into the maker. Cook for around 5 minutes and repeat with the rest of the batter.

32 Tasty Chaffles

(Ready in about 13 minutes | Serving 2 | Difficulty: Easy)

Per serving: Kcal 116, Fat: 9.5gg, Net Carbs: 2.6g, Protein: 4.5g

Ingredients

- 1 oz softened cream cheese
- 1 tbsp of almond flour
- 1 tbsp of pumpkin puree
- 1 egg
- 1/2 tsp of pumpkin spice

Instructions

Whisk the cream cheese in a bowl. Whisk pumpkin puree and egg in a bowl. Add almond flour and pumpkin spice and mix. Preheat the iron and spray using oil. Pour half amount of mixture in the maker and cook for around 5 minutes. Repeat with the rest of the batter.

33 Bread Sticks Chaffle

(Ready in about 12 minutes | Serving 7 | Difficulty: Easy)

Per serving: Kcal 80, Fat: 7g, Net Carbs: 1g, Protein: 5g

Ingredients

- 1 egg
- 2 tbsp of almond flour
- 1/2 cup grated mozzarella cheese
- 1/2tsp of garlic powder
- 1/2tsp of salt
- 1/2tsp of oregano

Topping

- 1/2tsp of garlic powder
- 2 tbsp softened butter
- 1/4 cup grated mozzarella cheese

Instructions

Preheat the maker and oil it. Mix all ingredients except topping ingredients. Pour in the maker and cook for around 5 minutes. Make four strips of waffle. Mix butter and garlic powder and coat strips with it. Sprinkle with mozzarella and cook for around 3 minutes.

34 Original Chaffle

(Ready in about 5 minutes | Serving 1 | Difficulty: Easy)

Per serving: Kcal 246, Fat: 18g, Net Carbs: 2g, Protein: 17g

Ingredients

- 2 eggs
- 1/4 cup of almond flour
- 1/2 cup of mozzarella
- 1/2 tsp of baking powder

Instructions

Preheat iron and spray with cooking spray. Mix all the ingredients in a bowl and pour half amount of the mixture into the maker. Cook for around 5 minutes and repeat with the rest of the mixture.

35 Mini Chaffles

(Ready in about 11 minutes | Serving 2 | Difficulty: Easy)

Per serving: Kcal 73, Fat: 6g, Net Carbs: 4g, Protein: 2g

Ingredients

- 2 tsp of Coconut Flour
- 1/4 tsp of Baking Powder
- 4 tsp of Swerve
- 1 Egg
- 1/2 tsp of Vanilla Extract
- 1 oz of Cream Cheese

Instructions

Preheat the iron. Add baking powder, coconut flour and swerve in a bowl and mix. Add cream cheese, egg and vanilla extract in bowl and mix. Pour mixture in the maker and cook for around 4 minutes.

36 Grain-free chaffles

(Ready in about 20 minutes | Serving 2 | Difficulty: Easy)

Per serving: Kcal 277, Fat: 20g, Net Carbs: 4.6g, Protein: 4.8g

Ingredients

- 1 tbsp of almond flour
- 1 tsp of vanilla
- 1 egg
- 1 shake of cinnamon
- 1 cup of mozzarella cheese
- 1 tsp of baking powder
- Butter

Instructions

Mix vanilla extract and egg in a bowl. Mix almond flour, baking powder and cinnamon. Add mozzarella cheese at the end and coat with the mixture evenly. Spray waffle using oil and turn it on. Pour mixture and cook for around 5 minutes. Top with butter and enjoy.

37 Healthy Chaffles

(Ready in about 20 minutes | Serving 4 | Difficulty: Easy)

Per serving: Kcal 411, Fat: 35g, Net Carbs: 6g, Protein: 21g

Ingredients

- 1 1/2 cup of shredded cheese cheddar
- 4 oz. cream cheese
- 4 eggs
- 2 tsp of baking powder
- 1/2 cup of almond flour
- Syrup

Instructions

Oil the waffle maker and mix all ingredients in a bowl. Pour batter into the maker and cook for around 5 minutes. Top with syrup(sugar-free) and enjoy.

38 Sunny Chaffle

(Ready in about 10 minutes | Serving 1 | Difficulty: Easy)

Per serving: Kcal 320, Fat: 24.3g, Net Carbs: 3.1g, Protein: 21.7g

Ingredients

- 1 egg
- Strawberries
- 2 tbsp of almond flour
- 1/2 cup of mozzarella cheese
- 1/2tsp of baking powder

Instructions

Preheat the maker and mix all the ingredients in a bowl. Pour into the center of the maker and cook for around 5 minutes. Top with strawberries and enjoy.

39 Traditional Chaffles

(Ready in about 13 minutes | Serving 1 | Difficulty: Easy)

Per serving: Kcal 291, Fat: 23g, Net Carbs: 1g, Protein: 20g

Ingredients

- 1/2 cup of shredded cheese cheddar
- 1 egg

Instructions

Preheat the maker and oil it gently. Break the egg in a bowl and add the half cup of cheddar cheese. Mix and pour half amount of mixture in maker. Cook for around 4 minutes. Repeat with the rest of the mixture.

40 Best Pizza Chaffle

(Ready in about 20 minutes | Serving 2 | Difficulty: Easy)

Per serving: Kcal 241, Fat: 18g, Net Carbs: 4g, Protein: 17g

Ingredients

- 1 tsp of coconut flour
- 1/2 cup of shredded cheese mozzarella
- 1 white of egg
- `1 tsp softened cream cheese
- 1/8 tsp of Italian seasoning
- 1/4 tsp of baking powder
- 1/8 tsp of garlic powder
- 3 tsp of marinara sauce
- Salt
- 1/2 cup of mozzarella cheese
- 1 tbsp shredded cheese parmesan
- 6 pepperonis diced in half
- 1/4 tsp of basil seasoning

Instructions

Preheat the oven to 400 degrees F. Preheat the maker as well. Add all the ingredients except pepperoni and parmesan cheese in a bowl and mix. Pour half amount of mixture in the maker and cook for around 4 minutes. Repeat with the rest of the mixture. Top with pepperoni, tomato sauce and parmesan cheese. Bake in the oven by placing on the top shelf for around 6 minutes. Turn broil setting and cook for around 2 minutes. Sprinkle with basil.

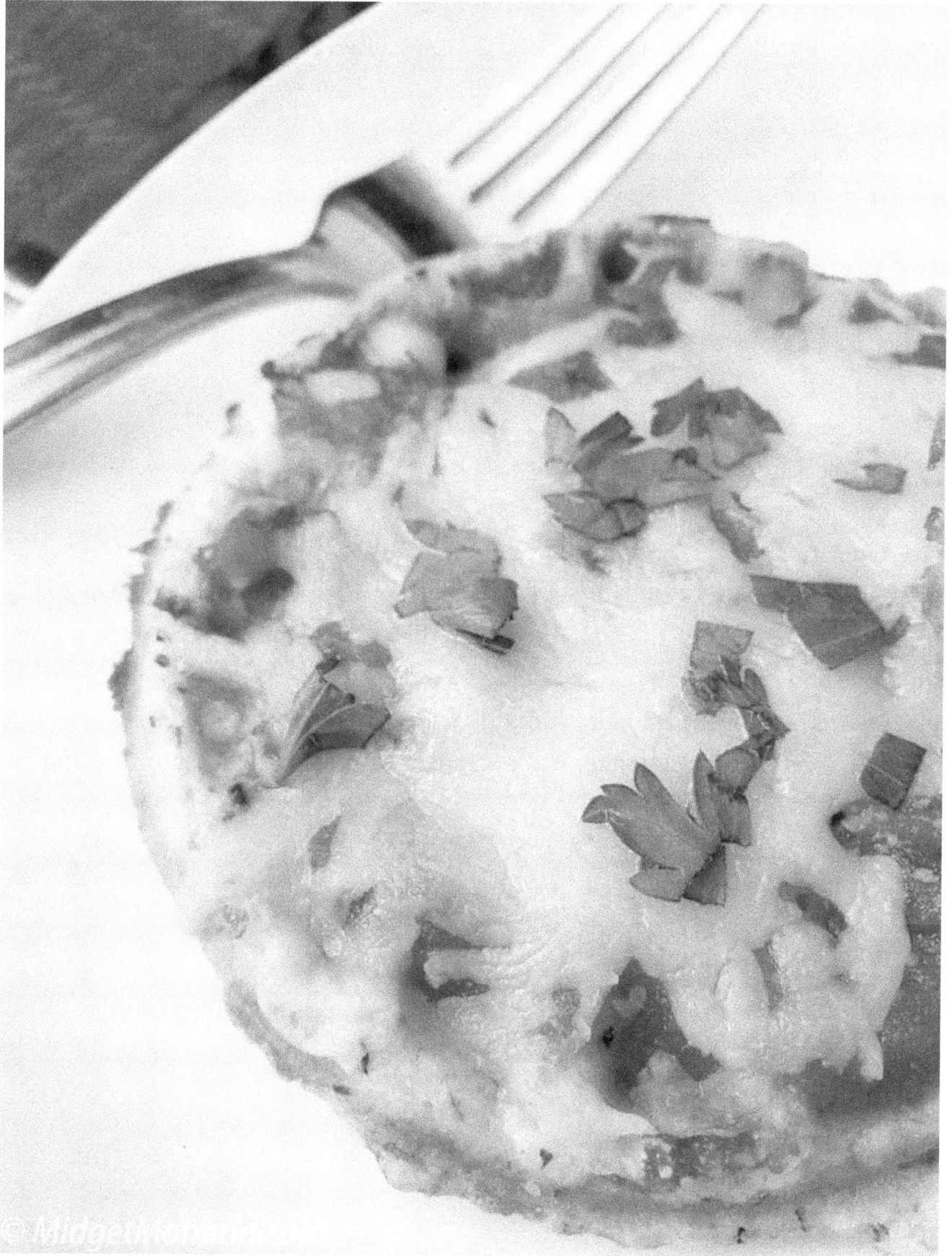

41 Open-Faced Chaffle

(Ready in about 17 minutes | Serving 2 | Difficulty: Easy)

Per serving: Kcal 118, Fat: 8g, Net Carbs: 2g, Protein: 9g

Ingredients

- 1 egg only white
- 1/4 cup shredded cheddar cheese
- 1/4 cup shredded cheese mozzarella
- 3/4 tsp of water
- 1/4 tsp of baking powder
- 1 tsp of coconut flour
- Salt

Instructions

Preheat the oven to 425 degrees F. Preheat the maker as well. Mix everything in a bowl and pour half the amount of mixture into a maker. Cook for around 4 minutes and repeat with the remaining mixture. Line parchment paper on a cookie sheet and place chaffles on it. Add a quarter cup of roasted keto beef gravy. Add cheese slice on top and bake in the oven for around 5 minutes in the top rack. Broil for around 1 minute.

42 Cream Chaffles

(Ready in about 15 minutes | Serving 2 | Difficulty: Easy)

Per serving: Kcal 293, Fat: 27g, Net Carbs: 5g, Protein: 10g

Ingredients

- 4 eggs
- 1 tsp of vanilla extract
- 2 tbsp of melted butter
- 4 oz of cream cheese
- 1 tsp of baking powder

Instructions

Blend all ingredients in a blender for around 1 minute. Spray the waffle maker using cooking spray and pour the mixture into the maker. Cook until it turns crispy and golden.

43 Fluffy Chaffles

(Ready in about 45 minutes | Serving 8 | Difficulty: Moderate)

Per serving: Kcal 140, Fat: 11g, Net Carbs: 4g, Protein: 4g

Ingredients

- 64 g of almond flour
- 1 1/2 tsp of baking powder
- 1 tbsp of ground psyllium husk
- 28 g of coconut flour
- 1 tsp of xanthan gum
- 57 g of butter
- 240 ml of water
- 3 tbsp of erythritol
- 3 eggs beaten
- 1/4 tsp of kosher salt
- 1 tsp of vanilla extract

Instructions

Mix flours, xantham gum and husk in a bowl. Warm water, sweetener, salt and butter in a pot and once it starts simmering, add flours and incorporate. Cook for around 3 minutes. Transfer dough to bowl and add egg one by one, mixing using an electric mixer. Add baking powder and vanilla extract and mix. Heat the maker and oil it. Pour batter and cook for around 12 minutes.

44 Almond Flour Chaffles

(Ready in about 20 minutes | Serving 2 | Difficulty: Easy)

Per serving: Kcal 70, Fat: 3.8g, Net Carbs: 4.9g, Protein: 4g

Ingredients

- 4 separated eggs
- 1/4 cup of granulated Swerve
- 2 cup of almond flour
- 2 tsp of baking powder
- 1/2 cup of butter
- 1 tsp of kosher salt
- 1/2 cup of almond butter
- Cooking spray
- 2 tsp. of vanilla extract
- Maple syrup

Instructions

Preheat waffle maker to high. Mix stevia, almond flour, salt and baking powder in a bowl. Melt almond butter and butter in the microwave for around 15 seconds. Stir dry ingredients with butter mixture and then add vanilla and yolks. Beat whites in a separate bowl and fold in batter. Spray maker using cooking spray and pour the batter. Cook for around 5 minutes. Top with maple syrup and butter.

45 Butter Chaffles

(Ready in about 30 minutes | Serving 5 | Difficulty: Easy)

Per serving: Kcal 216, Fat: 19.9g, Net Carbs: 5.5g, Protein: 6.4g

Ingredients

- 5 eggs
- 4 tbsp of granulated sweetener
- 4 tbsp of coconut flour
- 1 tsp of baking powder
- 3 tbsp of milk full fat
- 2 tsp of vanilla
- 125 g of butter melted

Instructions

Beat egg whites in a bowl. Mix yolks with sweetener, baking powder and coconut flour in a separate bowl. Add butter and mix. Add vanilla and milk and mix. Fold whites in yolk mixture and pour in maker. Cook for around 5 minutes.

46 Paleo Chaffles

(Ready in about 10minutes | Serving 2 | Difficulty: Easy)

Per serving: Kcal 401, Fat: 37, Net Carbs: 9g, Protein: 13g

Ingredients

- 1 egg
- 2 tbsp of sweetener
- 1/2 cup of Almond Flour
- 1/2 tsp of baking powder Gluten-free
- 2 tbsp of Almond butter
- 1/4 tsp of Sea salt
- 2 tbsp of Butter
- 1/2 tsp of Vanilla extract
- 1/4 cup of almond milk Unsweetened

Instructions

Preheat waffle maker to high temperature. Oil it gently and beat whites in a bowl. Combine baking powder, erythritol, salt and almond flour in another bowl. Melt almond butter and butter in the microwave and add to the flour mixture. Add yolk, vanilla and almond milk and stir. Fold whites in batter and mix. Pour in the maker and cook for around 5 minutes.

47 Crispy Chaffles

(Ready in about 10 minutes | Serving 4 | Difficulty: Easy)

Per serving: Kcal 64, Fat: 2g, Net Carbs: 4g, Protein: 5g

Ingredients

- 4 tbsp sifted coconut flour
- 1/4 tsp of baking powder
- 1 tsp of coconut oil
- 1 tbsp sweetener granulated
- 2/3 cup of egg whites
- 1/2 tsp of vanilla extract
- 1/4 cup of milk
- 1 tbsp of unsweetened apple sauce

Instructions

Mix sweetener, baking powder and coconut flour in a bowl. Add whites, vanilla, apple sauce and milk in a separate bowl and mix. Pour to the other bowl and form a thick batter. Add oil and spray waffle maker using cooking spray. Once the maker is hot, pour the batter and cook for around 4 minutes.

48 Salted Chaffles

(Ready in about 15 minutes | Serving 2 | Difficulty: Easy)

Per serving: Kcal 425, Fat: 36.7g, Net Carbs: 10.7g, Protein: 14.8g

Ingredients

Dry

- 3/4 cup of Almond Flour
- 1 tbsp of Coconut flour
- 2 tbsp of Erythritol
- 1 tsp of Baking Powder
- 1/8 tsp of Himalayan Salt

Wet

- 2 tbsp of Melted Butter
- 2 Eggs
- 2 tbsp of Cream Cheese at room temperature
- 1 tsp of Vanilla Extract

Instructions

Preheat waffle maker to high. Mix wet ingredients in a bowl. Mix dry ingredients in a separate bowl. Mix both bowls and pour in the maker. Cook for around 4 minutes.

49 Low Carb Chaffles

(Ready in about 8 minutes | Serving 1 | Difficulty: Easy)

Per serving: Kcal 522, Fat: 48g, Net Carbs: 7g, Protein: 19g

Ingredients

- 2 eggs
- 1/2 tsp of baking powder
- 4 tbsp of almond flour
- 2 oz of cream cheese
- 1 tbsp of coconut oil

Instructions

Blend everything in the blender and pour in the maker, which is oiled. Cook for around 3 minutes.

50 Sweet Chaffles

(Ready in about 9 minutes | Serving 2 | Difficulty: Easy)

Per serving: Kcal 331, Fat: 29g, Net Carbs: 7g, Protein: 11g

Ingredients

Dry

- 1/2 cup of almond flour
- 1/2 tsp of sweetener
- 1/4tsp of baking soda
- 1/4tsp of salt
- 1/4 tsp of baking powder
- 1/8 tsp of nutmeg
- 1/4tsp of ground cinnamon
- 1/8 tsp of cloves

Wet

- 2 eggs
- 2 tbsp of melted butter
- 1 tsp of vanilla extract

Instructions

Add dry ingredients to a bowl and mix. Separate yolks and whites in two bowls and mix butter and vanilla in yolks. Beat whites and add yolks to dry ingredients. Then add whites while mixing gently. Preheat maker to high temperature and pour the mixture. Cook for around 5 minutes.

51 Churro Chaffle

(Ready in about 15 minutes | Serving 1 | Difficulty: Easy)

Per serving: Kcal 193, Fat: 14g, Net Carbs: 2g, Protein: 8g

Ingredients

- 1 egg
- 1/4 cup of almond flour
- 1 tsp of cinnamon
- 1/2 cup of shredded cheese mozzarella
- 2 tbsp of Swerve granular
- 2 tbsp of melted butter
- ⅛ tsp of baking powder
- 3 tbsp of Swerve granular

Instructions

Combine everything in a bowl and pour the mixture into the maker by dividing it into three parts. Melt butter in the meantime in a pan over moderate flame. Add churro toppings and enjoy.

52 Avocado Egg Bake

(Ready in about 20 minutes | Serving 1 | Difficulty: Easy)

Per serving: Kcal 605, Fat: 50.9g, Net Carbs: 18.6g, Protein: 25.3g

Ingredients

- 2 eggs
- 1 avocado, pitted and halved
- ¼ cup of shredded Cheddar cheese
- 1 tbsp. chopped fresh parsley, or according to taste
- Freshly ground black pepper and salt according to taste

Instructions

- Preheat oven to 425 degrees Fahrenheit.
- To make way for one egg, scoop out some of the avocados from where the pit. Put each avocado half on the baking sheet, then crack one egg on top.
- Cook for fifteen to twenty minutes in a preheated oven before the egg is ready. Season with pepper and salt and finish with Cheddar cheese. Serve with new parsley as a garnish.

53 Oven-Baked Bacon

(Ready in about 35 minutes | Serving 6 | Difficulty: Easy)

Per serving: Kcal 134, Fat: 10.4g, Net Carbs: 0.4g, Protein: 9.2g

Ingredients

1 (16 oz.) package bacon

Instructions

- Preheat oven to 350°F. Using parchment paper, line a baking dish.
- Put the bacon slices on a prepared baking sheet, one on top of the other.
- Bake for fifteen to twenty minutes in a preheated oven. Take off the dish from the oven. Return the bacon slices to the oven after tossing them with kitchen tongs. Bake for another fifteen to twenty minutes, or till crispy. Thinner slices may require less time to cook, about twenty minutes overall. Drain on a paper towel-lined pan.

54 Roasted Leeks With Eggs

(Ready in about 40 minutes | Serving 2 | Difficulty: Easy)

Per serving: Kcal 1219, Fat: 124.6g, Net Carbs: 27.8g, Protein: 11.8g

Ingredients

- 3 green onions
- 2 leeks
- 2 tbsp. melted ghee (clarified butter)
- ¼ tsp. ground black pepper
- ½ tsp. sea salt

Avocado Vinaigrette:

- ¾ cup of light olive oil
- ⅛ tsp. red pepper flakes
- 1 ripe avocado, flesh scooped from the skin, pitted
- 1 lemon, juiced
- Ground black pepper and salt according to taste
- ¼ cup of red wine vinegar
- 1 tsp. olive oil
- ¼ cup of sliced, toasted almonds
- 2 eggs

Instructions

- Preheat oven to 400 degrees Fahrenheit.
- Green tops and bottom half-inch of the leeks should be discarded. Leeks can be sliced in half lengthwise.
- On a sheet tray, arrange the green onions and leeks. Drizzle ghee on top. Season with salt and pepper.
- For fifteen to twenty minutes in a preheated oven, roast till brown.
- In a food processor, thoroughly 3/4 cup olive oil, mix avocado, vinegar, lemon juice, pepper, and salt to make the vinaigrette

- In a skillet on medium-low flame, heat 1 tsp. oil for two to three minutes, or before whites are just set and the yolks are already runny, break eggs onto the opposite sides of the skillet.
- Remove the leeks and onions from the oven and put them on top with the sunny-side-up eggs. On top, sprinkle red pepper flakes and almonds. Finish with an avocado vinaigrette drizzle.

55 Gluten-Free Bagels

(Ready in about 30 minutes | Serving 6 | Difficulty: Easy)

Per serving: Kcal 364, Fat: 27.9g, Net Carbs: 9.7g, Protein: 20.9g

Ingredients

- 1 tbsp. baking powder, gluten-free
- 1 ½ cups of almond flour
- 2 eggs
- 1 tsp. garlic salt
- 2 oz. cream cheese, cubed
- 2 ½ cups of shredded mozzarella cheese

Instructions

- Preheat oven to 400 degrees Fahrenheit. Using parchment paper, line the baking sheet.
- In a mixing bowl, add the baking powder, garlic salt, and almond flour.
- In the microwave-safe bowl, mix mozzarella and cream cheese. Microwave for one minute, then remove and mix. Microwave for another minute, then take it off and stir until all is well combined. Working fast, stir the eggs and flour mixture into melted cheese mixture. Knead the dough by hand until it becomes a sticky dough. Continue kneading and pressing the dough for approximately two minutes or until it is fully uniform.
- The dough can be divided into six equal bits. Roll each one into the long log, then push the ends together to form a bagel shape and put it on the baking sheet that has been prepared.
- For ten to fourteen minutes in the preheated oven, bake till the bagels are golden.

55 Keto Zucchini Hash

(Ready in about 30 minutes | Serving 4 | Difficulty: Easy)

Per serving: Kcal 200, Fat: 17.9g, Net Carbs: 5g, Protein: g

Ingredients

- 3 tbsp. coconut oil
- 4 small zucchini, squeezed dry and grated
- 1 tbsp. butter
- 1 tsp. chili powder, or according to taste
- ⅓ cup of grated Parmesan cheese
- 1 tsp. sea salt
- 2 eggs, beaten
- 1 tsp. cayenne pepper (Optional)

Directions

- In a small skillet over medium flame, combine the coconut oil, butter, and zucchini. Add the chili powder, Parmesan cheese, cayenne pepper, and salt to a mixing bowl. Stir until the cheese has melted.
- Reduce the heat to a minimum and whisk in the eggs before thoroughly combined. Adjust to medium heat and fry, stirring and tossing sometimes, for almost fifteen minutes, or till the edges of hash are lightly browned.

Conclusion

A keto diet may be a healthier option for certain people, although the amount of fat, carbohydrates, and protein prescribed varies from person to person. If you have diabetes, talk to the doctor before starting the diet because it would almost certainly need prescription changes and stronger blood sugar regulation. Are you taking drugs for high blood pressure? Before starting a keto diet again, talk to the doctor. If you're breastfeeding, you shouldn't follow a ketogenic diet. Be mindful that limiting carbs will render you irritable, hungry, and sleepy, among other things. However, this may be a one-time occurrence. Keep in mind that you can eat a balanced diet in order to obtain all of the vitamins and minerals you need. A sufficient amount of fiber is also needed. When the body begins to derive energy from accumulated fat rather than glucose, it is said to be in ketosis. Several trials have shown the powerful weight-loss benefits of a low-carb, or keto, diet. This diet, on the other hand, can be difficult to stick to and can exacerbate health issues in individuals who have certain disorders, such as diabetes type 1. The keto diet is suitable for the majority of citizens. Nonetheless, all major dietary modifications should be discussed with a dietitian or doctor. This is essentially the case with people who have inherent conditions. The keto diet may be an effective therapy for people with drug-resistant epilepsy. Though the diet may be beneficial to people of any age, teenagers, people over 50, and babies can profit the most because they can easily stick to it. Modified keto diets, such as the revised Atkins diet or the low-glycemic index diet, are safer for adolescents and adults. A health care worker should keep a careful eye on someone who is taking a keto diet as a treatment. A doctor and dietitian will maintain track of a person's progress, administer drugs, and test for side effects. The body absorbs fat and protein differently than it does carbohydrates. Carbohydrates have a high insulin reaction. The protein sensitivity to insulin is mild, and the quick insulin response is negligible. Insulin is a fat-producing and fat-conserving enzyme. If you wish to lose weight, consume as many eggs, chickens, fish, and birds as you want, satiate yourself with the fat, and then eat every vegetable that grows on the ground. Butter and coconut oil can be used instead of processed synthetic seed oils. You may be either a sugar or a fat burner, but not both.

Healthy Keto Smoothies

A Complete Guide to get a Healthy keto Smoothies with step by step recipes to lose weight, promotes longevity and strengthen immune system.

By

Sonia Scott

Keto Smoothies And Shakes

1 Triple berry smoothie

(Ready in about 2 minutes | Serving 1 | Difficulty: Easy)

Per serving: Kcal 330, Fat: 26g, Net Carbs: 21g, Protein: 12g

Ingredients

- 2 tbsp of hemp seeds
- 1 cup of water
- Half avocado
- 1/2 cup of frozen berries (raspberries, blueberries, and strawberries)
- 2 cups of spinach

Instructions

Add everything to a blender and turn it on. Blend until smooth and enjoy.

2 Chocolate smoothie

(Ready in about 2 minutes | Serving 1 | Difficulty: Easy)

Per serving: Kcal 345, Fat: 31g, Net Carbs: 13g, Protein: 11

ingredients

- 1 cup of almond milk unsweetened
- 2 tbsp of peanut butter
- 1/4 cup of heavy cream
- 1 tbsp of cocoa powder unsweetened
- 1 cup of ice

Instructions

Add everything to a blender and turn it on. Blend until smooth and enjoy.

3 Zucchini smoothie

(Ready in about 2 minutes | Serving 1 | Difficulty: Easy)

Per serving: Kcal 219, Fat: 12g, Net Carbs: 24g, Protein: 7g

Ingredients

- 1 cup of zucchini chopped
- 1 cup of water
- 3 tbsp of chia seeds
- 1/2 cup of frozen strawberries

Instructions

Add everything to a blender and turn it on. Blend until smooth and enjoy.

4 Coconut smoothie

(Ready in about 2 minutes | Serving 1 | Difficulty: Easy)

Per serving: Kcal 321, Fat: 29g, Net Carbs: 17g, Protein: 4g

Ingredients

- 1/2 cup of full-fat unsweetened coconut milk
- 1/2 cup of blackberries frozen
- 10 mint leaves
- 2 tbsp of coconut shredded

Instructions

Add everything to a blender and turn it on. Blend until smooth and enjoy.

5 Lemon smoothie

(Ready in about 2 minutes | Serving 1 | Difficulty: Easy)

Per serving: Kcal 100, Fat: 6g, Net Carbs: 10g, Protein: 4g

Ingredients

- 1/2 cup of water
- 1 cup sliced cucumber
- 1/2 cup of ice
- 1 cup of spinach or kale
- 2 tbsp of flax seeds
- 1 tbsp of lemon juice

Instructions

Add everything to a blender and turn it on. Blend until smooth and enjoy.

6 Cinnamon smoothie

(Ready in about 2 minutes | Serving 1 | Difficulty: Easy)

Per serving: Kcal 286, Fat: 21g, Net Carbs: 19g, Protein: 10g

Ingredients

- 1 cup of almond milk unsweetened
- 1/8 tsp of cinnamon
- 1 cup of spinach
- 1/2 cup of raspberries frozen
- 2 tbsp of almond butter

Instructions

Add everything to a blender and turn it on. Blend until smooth and enjoy.

7 Strawberry smoothie

(Ready in about 2 minutes | Serving 1 | Difficulty: Easy)

Per serving: Kcal 431, Fat: 43g, Net Carbs: 10g, Protein: 4g

Ingredients

- 1/2 cup of water
- 1/2 cup of strawberries frozen
- 1/2 cup of heavy cream

Instructions

Add everything to a blender and turn it on. Blend until smooth and enjoy.

8 Cauliflower smoothie

(Ready in about 2 minutes | Serving 1 | Difficulty: Easy)

Per serving: Kcal 308, Fat: 23g, Net Carbs: 19g, Protein: 15g

Ingredients

- 1 cup of almond unsweetened
- 1 cup of cauliflower florets frozen
- 1.5 tbsp of cocoa powder unsweetened
- 1 tbsp of cacao nibs
- 3 tbsp of hemp seeds
- Sea salt

Instructions

Add everything to a blender and turn it on. Blend until smooth and enjoy.

Anyonita Nibbles

9 Pumpkin smoothie

(Ready in about 2 minutes | Serving 1 | Difficulty: Easy)

Per serving: Kcal 462, Fat: 42g, Net Carbs: 19g, Protein: 10g

Ingredients

- 1/2 cup of coconut milk unsweetened
- 1/2 cup of ice
- 2 tbsp of almond butter
- 1/2 cup of pumpkin purée
- 1/4 tsp of pie spice pumpkin
- Sea salt

Instructions

Add everything to a blender and turn it on. Blend until smooth and enjoy.

10 Lime pie smoothie

(Ready in about 2 minutes | Serving 1 | Difficulty: Easy)

Per serving: Kcal 281, Fat: 23g, Net Carbs: 17g, Protein: 8g

Ingredients

- 1 cup of water
- 1/4 cup of raw cashews
- 1/2 cup of almond milk unsweetened
- 1 cup of spinach
- 2 tbsp of lime juice
- 2 tbsp of coconut shredded

Instructions

Add everything to a blender and turn it on. Blend until smooth and enjoy.

11 Coconut Smoothie

(Ready in about 5 minutes | Serving 1 | Difficulty: Easy)

Per serving: Kcal 500, Fat: 38g, Net Carbs: 8g, Protein: 26g

Ingredients

- 3/4 cup canned coconut milk full-fat
- Handful of ice
- 2 tbsp cacao powder unsweetened
- 15 drops of liquid stevia coconut
- 2 scoops of collagen protein

Instructions

Add everything to the blender except collagen and turn it on. Blend until smooth and add collagen. Blend again and enjoy.

12 Cinnamon Smoothie

(Ready in about 5 minutes | Serving 1 | Difficulty: Easy)

Per serving: Kcal 300, Fat: 30g, Net Carbs: 14g, Protein: 3g

Ingredients

- 3/4 cup of coconut milk
- 2 tsp cacao powder unsweetened
- 1/2 ripe avocado
- 1 tsp of cinnamon powder
- Stevia
- 1/4 tsp of vanilla extract

Instructions

Add everything to a blender and turn it on. Blend until smooth and enjoy.

13 Avocado Smoothie

(Ready in about 5 minutes | Serving 1 | Difficulty: Easy)

Per serving: Kcal 552, Fat: 44g, Net Carbs: 10g, Protein: 26g

Ingredients

- 1/2 cup of coconut milk
- 2 tbsp of coconut shredded
- 1/2 cup of ice
- 1 cup of water
- 2 scoops of Collagen Protein Chocolate
- 4 mint leaves
- 1/2 cup of frozen avocado
- 1 tbsp of cacao butter crushed

Instructions

Add everything to the blender except coconut and turn it on. Blend until smooth and top with coconut and enjoy.

14 Keto Smoothie

(Ready in about 5 minutes | Serving 2 | Difficulty: Easy)

Per serving: Kcal 148, Fat: 11g, Net Carbs: 13g, Protein: 2g

Ingredients

- 1 cup of cold water
- 1/2 cup of cilantro
- 1 cup of baby spinach
- 1 inch peeled ginger
- 1/2-1 peeled lemon
- 3/4 English peeled cucumber
- 1 cup avocado frozen

Instructions

Add everything to a blender and turn it on. Blend until smooth and enjoy.

15 Cucumber Smoothie

(Ready in about 5 minutes | Serving 2 | Difficulty: Easy)

Per serving: Kcal 69, Fat: 4.6g, Net Carbs: 6.8g, Protein: 2g

Ingredients

- 8 ounces of water
- 1 cup cucumber sliced
- 2 tsp of Tea powder Match Green
- 2 ounces of ripe avocado
- 1/2 tsp of liquid stevia lemon
- 1 tsp of lemon juice
- 1/2 cup of ice

Instructions

Blend tea powder and water first, and then add the rest of the ingredients. Blend and enjoy.

16 Kale Shake

(Ready in about 5 minutes | Serving 1 | Difficulty: Easy)

Per serving: Kcal 141, Fat: 10.8g, Net Carbs: 8.6g, Protein: 4g

Ingredients

- 1 cup almond milk unsweetened
- 4 cups kale chopped
- 1/2 cup canned full-fat coconut milk
- 1/4 cup coconut ground
- 1/4 tsp of kosher salt
- 1 1-inch fresh ginger piece, peeled
- 1 cup of ice

Instructions

Add coconut milk first, and then almond, followed by the rest of the ingredients in a blender and turn it on. Blend until smooth and enjoy.

17 Turmeric Smoothie

(Ready in about 2 minutes | Serving 1 | Difficulty: Easy)

Per serving: Kcal 600, Fat: 56g, Net Carbs: 6g, Protein: 7g

Ingredients

- 200 ml coconut milk full fat
- 1 tbsp of Chia seeds
- 1 tsp of granulated sweetener
- 200 ml almond milk unsweetened
- 1 tbsp of ground turmeric
- 1 tsp of ground ginger
- 1 tsp of ground cinnamon
- 1 tbsp of MCT Oil

Instructions

Add everything except chia seeds to the blender and turn it on. Blend until smooth and top with seeds and enjoy.

18 Ginger Smoothie

(Ready in about 10 minutes | Serving 2 | Difficulty: Easy)

Per serving: Kcal 232, Fat: 22.4g, Net Carbs: 4.8g, Protein: 1.7g

Ingredients

- 1/2 avocado
- 1/4 cup of almond milk
- 3/4 cup coconut milk full - fat
- 1 tsp of grated ginger
- 1 tsp of lime juice
- 1/2 tsp of turmeric
- 1 cup of ice sweetener crushed

Instructions

Add everything except sweetener and ice to the blender and turn it on. Blend until smooth and add the rest of the ingredients and blend again.

19 Paleo Smoothie

(Ready in about 5 minutes | Serving 2 | Difficulty: Easy)

Per serving: Kcal 387, Fat: 25g, Net Carbs: 12g, Protein: 27g

Ingredients

- 1 cup of water
- stevia
- 1/2 cup of coconut milk full-fat
- 1 scraped gluten-free vanilla bean
- 2 tbsp of collagen hydrolysate
- 3 cups of ice
- 2 tbsp of golden flax ground

Instructions

Add everything to the blender and turn it on. Blend until smooth and enjoy.

20 Post Workout Smoothie

(Ready in about 3minutes | Serving 1 | Difficulty: Easy)

Per serving: Kcal 474, Fat: 21g, Net Carbs: 54g, Protein: 27g

Ingredients

- 1 cup full-fat coconut milk
- 2 cups of blueberries
- 3 tbsp of gelatin
- 2 cups of ice
- Stevia

Instructions

Add everything except gelatin to the blender and turn it on. Blend until smooth, and then add gelatin. Blend again and enjoy.

21 Dairy And Egg Free Smoothie

(Ready in about 5 minutes | Serving 2 | Difficulty: Easy)

Per serving: Kcal 288, Fat: 17g, Net Carbs: 10g, Protein: 14g

Ingredients

- 1 cup coconut milk full fat
- 1 13 oz can of pumpkin organic
- 1/2 tsp of powder extract stevia
- 1/2 cup of water
- 1 tsp of organic cinnamon
- 2-3 cups of ice cubes
- 2 tbsp of golden flax ground
- 2 tbsp of hydrolysate gelatin
- 1 tsp of cinnamon

Instructions

Add everything to the blender and turn it on. Blend until smooth and enjoy.

22 Chai Smoothie

(Ready in about 5 minutes | Serving 1 | Difficulty: Easy)

Per serving: Kcal 726, Fat: 69g, Net Carbs: 20g, Protein: 5.5g

Ingredients

- 3/4 cup of coconut milk full-fat
- 1/2tsp of pumpkin spice
- 1 tsp of chai tea
- 3 tbsp of pumpkin puree
- 1 tsp of vanilla
- 1/2 frozen avocado

Instructions

Add everything except avocado to the blender and turn it on. Blend until smooth and add avocado. Blend again and enjoy.

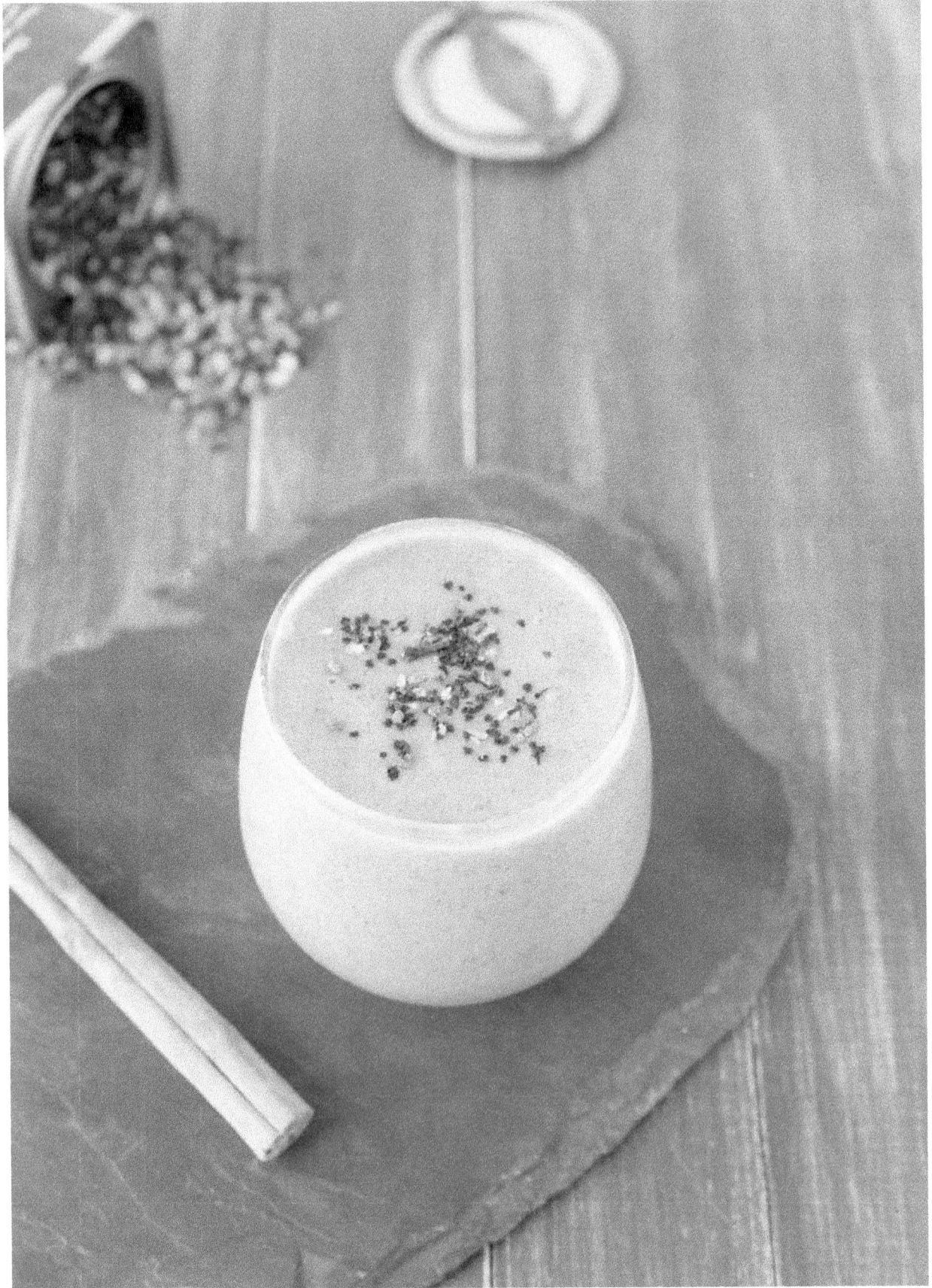

23 Raspberry Smoothie

(Ready in about 2 minutes | Serving 2 | Difficulty: Easy)

Per serving: Kcal 227, Fat: 20g, Net Carbs: 12.8g, Protein: 2.5g

Ingredients

- 1 ripe avocado pit removed and peeled
- 1 1/3 cup of water
- 2-3 tbsp of lemon juice
- 2 tbsp stevia extract
- 1/2 cup of frozen raspberries unsweetened

Instructions

Add everything to the blender and turn it on. Blend until smooth and enjoy.

24 Blueberry Smoothie

(Ready in about 5 minutes | Serving 1 | Difficulty: Easy)

Per serving: Kcal 215, Fat: 10g, Net Carbs: 7g, Protein: 23g

Ingredients

- 1 cup of Coconut Milk
- 1 tsp of Vanilla Extract
- 1/4 cup of Blueberries
- 1 tsp of MCT Oil

Instructions

Add everything to the blender and turn it on. Blend until smooth and enjoy.

25 Lime Strawberry Smoothie

(Ready in about 5 minutes | Serving 2 | Difficulty: Easy)

Per serving: Kcal 218, Fat: 13g, Net Carbs: 6g, Protein: 10g

Ingredients

- 1 can of coconut milk full fat
- 2 tbsp of MCT oil
- 8 ounces of frozen strawberries
- 1 tbsp freshly squeezed lime juice
- 1/4tsp of stevia
- 1 tbsp of lecithin powder

Instructions

Add everything to the blender and turn it on. Blend until smooth and enjoy.

26 Pie Smoothie

(Ready in about 5 minutes | Serving 2 | Difficulty: Easy)

Per serving: Kcal 753, Fat: 76g, Net Carbs: 20g, Protein: 14g

Ingredients

- 2 cups of coconut milk
- 4 tbsp of lime juice
- 2 tbsp of collagen
- 1/4 cup of macadamia nuts
- 1/2 medium-sized avocado
- 1 tbsp of erythritol
- 2 handfuls of spinach
- 2 tbsp of coconut butter
- One lime zest

Instructions

Add everything to the blender and turn it on. Blend until smooth and enjoy.

27 Base shake

(Ready in about 2 minutes | Serving 1 | Difficulty: Easy)

Per serving: Kcal 148, Fat: 10g, Net Carbs: 6g, Protein: 4g

Ingredients

- 1 cup almond milk unsweetened
- 1/2 cup of ice
- 2 tbsp of granulated sweetener
- 2 tbsp of almond butter

Instructions

Add everything to the blender and turn it on. Blend until smooth and enjoy.

28 Chocolate Shake

(Ready in about 2 minutes | Serving 1 | Difficulty: Easy)

Per serving: Kcal 148, Fat: 10g, Net Carbs: 6g, Protein: 4g

Ingredients

- 1/4 of avocado
- 2 tbsp of cocoa powder
- 1 cup almond milk unsweetened
- 1/2 cup of ice
- 2 tbsp of granulated sweetener
- 2 tbsp of almond butter

Instructions

Add everything to the blender and turn it on. Blend until smooth and enjoy.

29 Vanilla Shake

(Ready in about 2 minutes | Serving 1 | Difficulty: Easy)

Per serving: Kcal 148, Fat: 10g, Net Carbs: 6g, Protein: 4g

Ingredients

- 1/4 cup of frozen cauliflower
- 1 tsp of vanilla extract
- 1 cup almond milk unsweetened
- 1/2 cup of ice
- 2 tbsp of granulated sweetener
- 2 tbsp of almond butter

Instructions

Add everything to the blender and turn it on. Blend until smooth and enjoy.

30 Strawberry Shake

(Ready in about 2 minutes | Serving 1 | Difficulty: Easy)

Per serving: Kcal 148, Fat: 10g, Net Carbs: 6g, Protein: 4g

Ingredients

- 1/4 cup of frozen strawberries
- 1 tsp of vanilla extract
- 1 cup almond milk unsweetened
- 1/2 cup of ice
- 2 tbsp of granulated sweetener
- 2 tbsp of almond butter

Instructions

Add everything to the blender and turn it on. Blend until smooth and enjoy.

31 Blueberry Shake

(Ready in about 2 minutes | Serving 1 | Difficulty: Easy)

Per serving: Kcal 148, Fat: 10g, Net Carbs: 6g, Protein: 4g

Ingredients

- 1/4 cup of frozen blueberries
- 1 tsp of vanilla extract
- 1 cup almond milk unsweetened
- 1/2 cup of ice
- 2 tbsp of granulated sweetener
- 2 tbsp of almond butter

Instructions

Add everything to the blender and turn it on. Blend until smooth and enjoy.

32 Cinnamon Shake

(Ready in about 2 minutes | Serving 1 | Difficulty: Easy)

Per serving: Kcal 148, Fat: 10g, Net Carbs: 6g, Protein: 4g

Ingredients

- 1 tbsp of cinnamon
- 1 tsp of vanilla extract
- 1/4 cup of frozen cauliflower
- 1 cup almond milk unsweetened
- 1/2 cup of ice
- 2 tbsp of granulated sweetener
- 2 tbsp of almond butter

Instructions

Add everything to the blender and turn it on. Blend until smooth and enjoy.

33 Base Shake 2

(Ready in about 5 minutes | Serving 1 | Difficulty: Easy)

Ingredients

- 1 cup of Almond Milk
- 1 tbsp of Almond Butter
- 1/2 cup of ice
- 2 tbsp of Whipping Cream

Instructions

Add everything to the blender and turn it on. Blend until smooth and enjoy.

34 Lemon Shake

(Ready in about 5 minutes | Serving 1 | Difficulty: Easy)

Per serving: Kcal 354, Fat: 32.2g, Net Carbs: 11.3g, Protein: 8.1g

Ingredients

- 1/4 cup of Frozen Blueberries
- 5 drops of Liquid Stevia
- 1 tsp of Lemon Juice
- 2 tbsp of Cream Cheese
- 1/4 tsp of Lemon Zest
- 1 cup of Almond Milk
- 1 tbsp of Almond Butter
- 1/2 cup of ice
- 2 tbsp of Whipping Cream

Instructions

Add everything to the blender with base ingredients and turn it on. Blend until smooth and enjoy.

35 Pumpkin Spice Shake

(Ready in about 5 minutes | Serving 1 | Difficulty: Easy)

Per serving: Kcal 335, Fat: 30.6g, Net Carbs: 10.2g, Protein: 9.9g

Ingredients

- 2 tbsp of Pumpkin Puree
- 1 pinch of Grated Nutmeg
- 1/4 tsp of Pumpkin Pie Spice
- 1 tbsp of Almond Butter
- 5-10 drops of Liquid Stevia
- 1 cup of Almond Milk
- 1 tbsp of Almond Butter
- 1/2 cup of ice
- 2 tbsp of Whipping Cream

Instructions

Add everything with base ingredients to the blender and turn it on. Blend until smooth and enjoy.

36 Peanut Butter Shake

(Ready in about 5 minutes | Serving 1 | Difficulty: Easy)

Per serving: Kcal 419, Fat: 32.9g, Net Carbs: 10.9g, Protein: 23.5g

Ingredients

- 1/2 scoop of Protein Powder Chocolate
- 1 tbsp of Peanut Butter
- 1 tsp of Cocoa Powder Unsweetened
- 5-10 drops of Liquid Stevia
- 1 dark chocolate Square
- 1 cup of Almond Milk
- 1 tbsp of Almond Butter
- 1/2 cup of ice
- 2 tbsp of Whipping Cream

Instructions

Add everything to the blender except chocolate squares with base ingredients and turn it on. Blend until smooth and top with squares and enjoy.

37 Tiramisu Shake

(Ready in about 5 minutes | Serving 1 | Difficulty: Easy)

Per serving: Kcal 381, Fat: 35.8g, Net Carbs: 9.5g, Protein: 8.4g

Ingredients

- 1 Shot of coffee espresso
- 1 tsp of Cocoa Powder Unsweetened
- 2 tbsp of Cream Cheese
- 1 dark chocolate Square
- 5-10 drops of Liquid Stevia
- 1 cup of Almond Milk
- 1 tbsp of Almond Butter
- 1/2 cup of ice
- 2 tbsp of Whipping Cream

Instructions

Add everything to the blender except chocolate squares with base ingredients and turn it on. Blend until smooth and enjoy.

38 Birthday Cake

(Ready in about 5 minutes | Serving 1 | Difficulty: Easy)

Per serving: Kcal 414, Fat: 36.2g, Net Carbs: 8g, Protein: 18.1g

Ingredients

- 1/2 scoop of Protein Powder Vanilla
- 1 tsp of Sprinkles Sugar-Free
- 1/4 tsp of Almond extract
- 1 tbsp of Melted Butter
- 5-10 drops of Liquid Stevia
- 1 cup of Almond Milk
- 1 tbsp of Almond Butter
- 1/2 cup of ice
- 2 tbsp of Whipping Cream

Instructions

Add everything to the blender except half amount of sprinkles with base ingredients and turn it on. Blend until smooth and top with sprinkles and enjoy.

39 Shamrock Shake

(Ready in about 5 minutes | Serving 1 | Difficulty: Easy)

Per serving: Kcal 259, Fat: 14g, Net Carbs: 7g, Protein: 26g

Ingredients

- 1/2 medium-sized avocado
- 1 scoop of protein powder vanilla
- 1/2 cup of almond
- 8 ice cubes
- ⅛ tsp of peppermint extract
- 5 drops of natural food coloring green
- 1 tbsp of chocolate chips dark

Instructions

Add everything except chocolate chips to the blender and turn it on. Blend until smooth and top using chocolate chips and enjoy.

40 Coconut Shake

(Ready in about 5 minutes | Serving 2 | Difficulty: Easy)

Per serving: Kcal 222, Fat: 23.1g, Net Carbs: 5.4g, Protein: 2.5g

Ingredients

- 4 oz full-fat coconut cream
- 8 oz almond
- 1/2 tbsp of almond butter
- 2 tbsp of coconut oil
- Sea salt
- 2 tbsp of cocoa powder

Instructions

Add everything to the blender and turn it on. Blend until smooth and enjoy.

41 Peppermint Milkshake

(Ready in about 5 minutes | Serving 1 | Difficulty: Easy)

Per serving: Kcal 436, Fat: 42g, Net Carbs: 15g, Protein: 5g

Ingredients

- 8 ounces of coconut cream
- 1/4 cup of organic spinach
- 2 tbsp of cocoa powder
- 1/2 tsp of stevia glycerite
- 2 drops of peppermint extract
- 1 cup of almond milk unsweetened
- 1 pinch of Himalayan salt

Instructions

Add everything to the blender and turn it on. Blend until smooth and enjoy.

42 Strawberry Milkshake

(Ready in about 5 minutes | Serving 1 | Difficulty: Easy)

Per serving: Kcal 276, Fat: 27.4g, Net Carbs: 6.4g, Protein: 2.5g

Ingredients

- 1/4 cup of coconut milk
- 1 tbsp of MCT oil
- 1/2 cup of strawberries
- 3/4 cup of almond milk unsweetened
- 1/2 tsp of vanilla extract sugar-free

Instructions

Add everything to the blender and turn it on. Blend until smooth and enjoy.

43 Blackberry Shake

(Ready in about 3 minutes | Serving 1 | Difficulty: Easy)

Per serving: Kcal 364, Fat: 34g, Net Carbs: 4.8g, Protein: 2.6g

Ingredients

- 7 cubes of ice
- 2 tbsp of MCT oil
- 1/4 cup of blackberries
- 1 cup of coconut milk unsweetened
- 2 tbsp of cocoa powder
- 1/4tsp of xanthan gum
- 12 drops of liquid stevia

Instructions

Add everything to the blender and turn it on. Blend until smooth and enjoy.

44 Frozen Berry Shake

(Ready in about 5 minutes | Serving 1 | Difficulty: Easy)

Per serving: Kcal 400, Fat: 41g, Net Carbs: 6.7g, Protein: 4g

Ingredients

- 1/3 cup of coconut milk
- Ice cubes
- 1/2 cup of frozen berries
- 1/2 cup of water
- 1 tbsp of MCT oil

Instructions

Place coconut milk in the fridge overnight to cream it. Extract solidified milk from the can and add the rest of the ingredients to the blender and turn it on. Blend until smooth and enjoy.

45 Cookies Milkshake

(Ready in about 15 minutes | Serving 2 | Difficulty: Easy)

Per serving: Kcal 546, Fat: 50g, Net Carbs: 8g, Protein: 5g

Ingredients

For crumbs

- 1 tbsp of butter melted
- 30 g of almond flour
- 1-2 tbsp of powdered erythritol
- 6 g of cocoa powder
- Kosher salt

For milkshake

- 1/4 cup of almond milk unsweetened
- 2 cups of ice cream vanilla

Instructions

For crumbs

Toast flour in a pan for around 4 minutes. Transfer to a bowl and mix with the rest of the oreo ingredients. Place in freezer.

For milkshake

Add everything with the half-crumbs mixture to the blender and turn it on. Blend until smooth and add the rest of the crumbs and enjoy.

46 Batter Milkshake

(Ready in about 2 minutes | Serving 1 | Difficulty: Easy)

Per serving: Kcal 480, Fat: 46.4g, Net Carbs: 7.95g, Protein: 15.98g

Ingredients

- 1/2 cup of almond milk
- 1/4 cup of crushed ice
- 1/4 cup of coconut milk full fat
- 50g of ground almonds
- 7 drops of liquid stevia
- 1 tsp of coconut oil
- 1/4 tsp of vanilla powder

Instructions

Add everything to the blender and turn it on. Blend until smooth and enjoy.

47 Cookie Milkshake

(Ready in about 1 hour 10 minutes | Serving 1 | Difficulty: Easy)

Per serving: Kcal 120, Fat: 2.5g, Net Carbs: 25g, Protein: 2g

Ingredients

- 3 cups of milk
- 1/2 tsp of vanilla extract
- 1/4 tsp of baking soda
- 1 frozen banana
- 1/4 tsp of tartar cream

Instructions

Add everything to the blender and turn it on. Blend until smooth and enjoy.

48 Almond Butter Shake

(Ready in about 2 minutes | Serving 1 | Difficulty: Easy)

Per serving: Kcal 326, Fat: 27g, Net Carbs: 11g, Protein: 19g

Ingredients

- 1 1/2 cups of nut milk unsweetened
- 2 Tbsp of almond butter
- 1/8 tsp of salt
- 1 scoop of collagen peptides
- 2 Tbsp of golden flax meal
- 15 drops of liquid stevia
- 1/2 tsp of cinnamon
- 1/8 tsp of almond extract
- 6 ice cubes

Instructions

Add everything to the blender and turn it on. Blend until smooth and enjoy.

49 Turmeric Milkshake

(Ready in about 5 minutes | Serving 1 | Difficulty: Easy)

Per serving: Kcal 351, Fat: 35.2g, Net Carbs: 6.9g, Protein: 1.6g

Ingredients

- 375 ml of coconut milk
- 3/4 tsp of turmeric powder
- Himalayan salt
- 2 tbsp of coconut oil
- 1/2 tsp of ginger powder
- 1/4 tsp of vanilla
- 1/4 tsp of cinnamon
- granulated sweetener
- 2 ice cubes

Instructions

Add everything to the blender and turn it on. Blend until smooth and enjoy.

50 Cinnamon Roll Shake

(Ready in about 5 minutes | Serving 1 | Difficulty: Easy)

Per serving: Kcal 386, Fat: 17g, Net Carbs: 8g, Protein: 12g

Ingredients

- 1 cup of almond milk
- 1 tsp of cinnamon
- 2 Tbsp of almond butter
- 1/4 tsp of vanilla
- 1/4 cup of ice cubes
- 1 Tbsp of Liquid Sweetener
- 1 scoop of Powdered Collagen
- 1 dash of nutmeg

Instructions

Add everything to the blender and turn it on. Blend until smooth and enjoy.

51 Hot Chocolate Shake

(Ready in about 8 minutes | Serving 4 | Difficulty: Easy)

Per serving: Kcal 770, Fat: 40g, Net Carbs: 89, Protein: 12g

Ingredients

- 1 1/2 cups of almond milk unsweetened
- 1 tsp of liquid stevia
- 1/2 cup of protein powder chocolate
- 3 ounces of chocolate chopped
- 1/2 tsp of peppermint extract
- 2 cups of ice

Instructions

Add everything to the blender and turn it on. Blend until smooth and enjoy.

Chocolate Milkshake

52 Bacon Milkshake

(Ready in about 5 minutes | Serving 1 | Difficulty: Easy)
Per serving: Kcal 386, Fat: 17g, Net Carbs: 8g, Protein: 12g

The shake

- 6 Tbsp of heavy cream
- 4 Tbsp of bacon fat
- 4 Tbsp of maple syrup
- 10 scoops of ice cream vanilla

The syrup

- 4 Tbsp of replacement brown sugar
- 4 Tbsp of cocoa
- 4 Tbsp of butter

The cream

- 1/4 tsp of maple extract
- 1 cup of white cream
- 1/4 cup of sweetener

Instructions

Whip maple extract, sweetener and heavy cream in a bowl for around 5 minutes. Add the rest of the ingredients to the blender and turn it on. Blend until smooth and top with whipped cream. Heat syrup ingredients in the microwave for around 20 seconds and drizzle on shake.

53 Homemade Milk

(Ready in about 9Hrs 5 minutes | Serving 4 | Difficulty: medium)
Per serving: Kcal 176, Fat: 13g, Net Carbs: 11.5g, Protein: 5.7g

Ingredients

- ⅓ cup of skin-on, raw almonds
- ⅓ cup of rolled oats
- 1 tbsp. whole flax seeds
- 4 cup of filtered water, divided
- ⅓ cup of cashews

Directions

- In a large mixing bowl, add the almonds, cashews, and oats and fill with 2 cups of water. Allow at least eight hours to absorb in the refrigerator.
- Remove from the refrigerator and stir in the flax seeds. Allow 1 hour for the flax seeds to interact with water and the mixture to hit room temperature.
- Blend until smooth and creamy in a blender. Allow for five-minute to rest. Add the last two cups of filtered water. Blend till smooth, creamy, and well mixed. Using a fine-mesh sieve, filter the pulp. You should eat it straight away or keep it in the fridge for up to a week, until using, giving it a good shake.

54 Vanilla Almond Shake

(Ready in about 5 minutes | Serving 1 | Difficulty: Easy)

Per serving: Kcal 176, Fat: 13g, Net Carbs: 11.5g, Protein: 5.7g

Ingredients

- 1 tbsp. sliced almonds
- ½ cup of ice
- 1 cup of water
- 1 tsp. sugar-free, Fats-free, vanilla pudding mix
- ⅔ cup of powdered milk, non-Fat

Directions

- Blend ice, 1/4 cup water, and almonds in a blender till the almonds are pulverized. Add the remaining powdered milk, pudding mix, and water, then continue blending till smooth.

55 Complete Breakfast Smoothie

(Ready in about 5 minutes | Serving 1 | Difficulty: Easy)

Per serving: Kcal 362, Fat: 9.4g, Net Carbs:45.1g, Protein: 28.2g

Ingredients

- ½ cup of berries, mixed frozen
- ¼ cup of Greek yogurt
- ¼ cup of oats, steel-cut
- ¼ cup of water
- 1 scoop of protein powder
- 1 tsp of honey

Directions

- In a processor, mix berries, yogurt, protein powder, oats, water, & honey until smooth.
- Chef's Notes: You may substitute flavored yogurt for plain yogurt. Simply keep an eye on the sugar level while you're monitoring the glucose intake.
- This is a good source of protein which fiber & will keep you going until lunch.
- Utilize whichever sweetener you want in the proportions that complement your palate. In this dish, sugar, Splenda(R), honey, and stevia all fit well.
- If you like, you may also use a protein powder that is flavored.
- You will adjust the berry mix to your preference. In every mix, blend strawberries, raspberries, blueberries, blackberries, & cherries.

56 Grapefruit, Lime & Mint Yogurt Parfait

(Ready in about 15 minutes | Serving 6 | Difficulty: Easy)

Per serving: Kcal 207, Fat: 3g, Net Carbs:39g, Protein: 10g

Ingredients

- 4 large grapefruit red
- 4 cups of plain yogurt reduced fat
- 2 tsp lime zest grated
- 2 tbsp lime juice
- 3 tbsp honey
- mint leaves, Torn fresh

Directions:

- Every grapefruit should have a tiny slice cut from the top & bottom; put fruit upright over the cutting board. Remove the outer membrane and peel from the grapefruit using a knife. Remove fruit by cutting along the surface of each segment.
- Combine lime zest, yogurt, and juice in a mixing cup. In six parfait glasses, layer grapefruit & yogurt mixture. Repetition of layers. Drizzle honey over the top; garnish with mint.

Conclusion

A keto diet may be a healthier option for certain people, although the amount of fat, carbohydrates, and protein prescribed varies from person to person. If you have diabetes, talk to the doctor before starting the diet because it would almost certainly need prescription changes and stronger blood sugar regulation. Are you taking drugs for high blood pressure? Before starting a keto diet again, talk to the doctor. If you're breastfeeding, you shouldn't follow a ketogenic diet. Be mindful that limiting carbs will render you irritable, hungry, and sleepy, among other things. However, this may be a one-time occurrence. Keep in mind that you can eat a balanced diet in order to obtain all of the vitamins and minerals you need. A sufficient amount of fiber is also needed. When the body begins to derive energy from accumulated fat rather than glucose, it is said to be in ketosis. Several trials have shown the powerful weight-loss benefits of a low-carb, or keto, diet. This diet, on the other hand, can be difficult to stick to and can exacerbate health issues in individuals who have certain disorders, such as diabetes type 1. The keto diet is suitable for the majority of citizens. Nonetheless, all major dietary modifications should be discussed with a dietitian or doctor. This is essentially the case with people who have inherent conditions. The keto diet may be an effective therapy for people with drug-resistant epilepsy. Though the diet may be beneficial to people of any age, teenagers, people over 50, and babies can profit the most because they can easily stick to it. Modified keto diets, such as the revised Atkins diet or the low-glycemic index diet, are safer for adolescents and adults. A health care worker should keep a careful eye on someone who is taking a keto diet as a treatment. A doctor and dietitian will maintain track of a person's progress, administer drugs, and test for side effects. The body absorbs fat and protein differently than it does carbohydrates. Carbohydrates have a high insulin reaction. The protein sensitivity to insulin is mild, and the quick insulin response is negligible. Insulin is a fat-producing and fat-conserving enzyme. If you wish to lose weight, consume as many eggs, chickens, fish, and birds as you want, satiate yourself with the fat, and then eat every vegetable that grows on the ground. Butter and coconut oil can be used instead of processed synthetic seed oils. You may be either a sugar or a fat burner, but not both.